MW01234336

Regional Anesthesia for Cardiothoracic Surgery

Edited by
Mark A. Chaney, M.D.

Associate Professor
Department of Anesthesia and Critical Care
Associate Director, Cardiac Anesthesia
University of Chicago
Chicago, Illinois

With 10 contributors

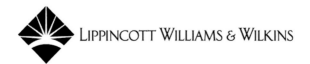 LIPPINCOTT WILLIAMS & WILKINS

Regional Anesthesia for Cardiothoracic Surgery

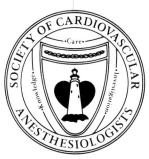

A Society of
Cardiovascular Anesthesiologists
Monograph

Copyright © 2002
SOCIETY OF CARDIOVASCULAR ANESTHESIOLOGISTS

All rights reserved. This book is protected by copyright. No part of this book
may be Reproduced in any form or by any means, including photocopying, or
utilized by any Information storage and retrieval system without written permission from the copyright owner.

Accurate indications, adverse reactions, and dosage schedules for drugs are provided in this
book, but it is possible that they may change. The reader is urged to review the package information data of the manufacturers of the medications mentioned.

Printed in the United States of America
(ISBN 0-781-73761-3)

02 03 04 05 06
1 2 3 4 5 6 7 8

Publication Committee of the
Society of Cardiovascular Anesthesiologists

Jeffrey R. Balser, M.D., Ph.D.
Nashville, Tennessee

Elliott Bennett-Guerrero, M.D.
New York, New York

Mark A. Chaney, M.D.
Chicago, Illinois

David J. Cook, M.D.
Rochester, Minnesota

Jean Yves Dupuis, M.D.
Ottawa, Ontario, Canada

Patricia M. Gramling-Babb, M.D.
Chicago, Illinois

Tim Grayson
Baltimore, Maryland

Joseph P. Mathew, M.D.
Durham, North Carolina

Johanna C. Schwarzenberger, M.D.
New York, New York

Preface

Regional anesthetic techniques (primarily intrathecal and epidural) are being utilized with increasing frequency by anesthesiologists managing patients undergoing cardiothoracic surgery. Potential perioperative benefits of regional anesthetic techniques (either alone or supplementing general anesthesia) include intense postoperative analgesia, stress response attenuation, and/or thoracic cardiac sympathectomy. However, potential risks exist when utilizing regional anesthetic techniques. The most feared risk is hematoma formation, especially when one considers the fact that most patients undergoing cardiothoracic surgery are subjected to some degree of perioperative anticoagulation. As always, when applying any specific intervention to any individual patient, potential benefits must be weighed against potential risks. This Society of Cardiovascular Anesthesiologists Monograph presents the potential benefits and potential risks of utilizing regional anesthetic techniques in patients undergoing cardiothoracic surgery.

Contributors

Mark A. Chaney, M.D.
Associate Professor
Department of Anesthesia and
    Critical Care
Associate Director, Cardiac
    Anesthesia
University of Chicago
Chicago, Illinois

**Oscar A. de Leon-Casasola,
    M.D.**
Professor of Anesthesiology
Vice-Chair for Clinical Affairs
University at Buffalo
School of Medicine
Buffalo, New York

**Étienne de Médicis, M. Sc.,
    M.D., F.R.C.P.(C)**
Adjunct Professor
Department of Anesthesiology
University of Sherbrook
Sherbrook, Quebec, Canada

John E. Ellis, M.D.
Professor
Department of Anesthesia and
    Critical Care
The University of Chicago
Chicago, Illinois

Gregory B. Hammer, M.D.
Associate Professor
Department of Anesthesiology and
    Pediatrics
Stanford University
Stanford, California

Terese T. Horlocker, M.D.
Associate Professor
Department of Anesthesiology
Mayo Clinic
Rochester, Minnesota

James F. McKinsey, M.D.
Associate Professor
Department of Surgery
The University of Chicago
Chicago, Illinois

**Karen McRae, M.D.C.M.,
    F.R.C.P.(C)**
Assistant Professor
Department of Anesthesia
University of Toronto
Toronto General Hospital
Toronto, Ontario, Canada

Norbert Rolf, M.D., Ph.D.
Department of Anesthesiology and
    Intensive Care Medicine
University Hospital
Muenster, Germany

Peter D. Slinger, M.D.,
  F.R.C.P.(C)
Professor
Department of Anesthesia
University of Toronto
Toronto General Hospital
Toronto, Ontario, Canada

Contents

Étienne de Médicis, M. Sc., M.D., F.R.C.P.(C)
Oscar A. de Leon-Casasola, M.D.

1 | Recent Advances in Regional Anesthesia

INTRODUCTION

A recent review of published randomized trials of intraoperative neur-axial blockade revealed substantial benefits in favor of the use of re-gional anesthesia, which reduced mortality by one-third (1). Moreover, neuraxial blockade was also associated with a reduced incidence of deep vein thrombosis, pulmonary embolism, transfusion requirement, pneumonia, respiratory depression, myocardial infarction, and renal failure. This investigation, as well as others, has generated a renewed interest in the benefits of regional anesthesia. Thus, new agents are under development, and regional anesthesia techniques are being refined.

THE NEW LOCAL ANESTHETICS

Bupivacaine is probably the most commonly utilized local anesthetic and has been tested in multiple clinical investigations. It is a long-acting agent that is commonly used for infiltration, nerve block, and spinal and/or epidural anesthesia and analgesia (in both obstetrical and nonobstetrical settings). It is an amide-type local anesthesic with a butyl side chain and is a racemic mixture of two enantiomers: R(+) and S(−). The safety of bupivacaine has been well documented in the perioperative setting (2–4). Conversely, inadvertent intravenous injections of bupivacaine have been associated with cardiac arrest and death (5, 6). Nonetheless, a

Regional Anesthesia for Cardiothoracic Surgery, edited by Mark Chaney, Lippincott Williams & Wilkins, Baltimore © 2002.

recent prospective study of French regional anesthesia practice documented 14 seizures due to bupivacaine injection with no associated cardiac arrest, suggesting that practitioners may be beneficially adjusting their regional anesthetic techniques (7). Moreover, since the Food and Drug Administration withdrew its approval for epidural administration of 0.75% bupivacaine in obstetric patients in 1984, there has been a decrease in reported maternal death from local anesthetic toxicity (8).

Bupivacaine binds to sodium channels rapidly, yet unbinds slowly, allowing the potential for a high fraction of sodium channels to be blocked (9). The blockade of the sodium channels leads to myocardial conduction block (increased PR and QRS intervals) (10). At higher concentrations, local anesthetics block potassium and calcium channels, leading to decreased inotropy, conduction block, and pulseless electrical activity (11–13). At even higher concentrations, beyond those needed to cause cardiac arrest due to blockade of sodium and calcium channels, there is RYR2-calcium channel blockade, beta-2 adrenergic receptor blockade, and mitochondrial metabolism inhibition, explaining the difficulty in resuscitating patients with bupivacaine-induced cardiac toxicity (14–16).

Multiple studies have demonstrated the decreased cardiotoxic properties of lidocaine when compared to bupivacaine, yet its shorter duration of action may limit its clinical use (17–20). This fact has stimulated research into developing less cardiotoxic local anesthetics. The presence of chirality (a chiral carbon is one in which the four bonding atoms or groups of atoms are different) within local anesthetics led to the potential for a molecule to exist in two different, three-dimensional, mirror-imaged, configurations: the S [left] and L [right]. Research involving new local anesthetic molecules and chirality has developed new drugs that are long-acting and have less cardiotoxicity than bupivacaine. It appears that S(−) enantiomers are less cardiotoxic because of the preferential binding of the R(+) enantiomer to cardiac sodium channels. The fruits of this research are ropivacaine (the S(−) enantiomer of an amide local anesthetic with a propyl side chain) and levobupivacaine (the S(−) enantiomer of bupivacaine).

Ropivacaine

The physicochemical properties of ropivacaine are essentially the same as bupivacaine except for lipid solubility (assessed via the octanol/buffer partition coefficient) (see Table 1–1). The onset of action (related to pKa) and duration of action (related to protein binding) of the two drugs are equivalent. The difference between the two drugs regarding lipid solubility implies that bupivacaine is a more potent drug than ropi-

TABLE 1–1. Physicochemical Properties of Local Anesthetics

Physicochemical properties	R(+) bupivacaine	S(−) bupivacaine	S(−) ropivacaine
Molecular weight	288	288	274
pKa	8.2	8.2	8.2
Ocatnol/buffer coefficient	346	346	115
Protein binding (%)	96	96	94

vacaine in vivo. This also explains, at least in part, why ropivacaine is less cardiotoxic than bupivacaine. The less lipid soluble a drug is, the less likely it is to enter the cell and be available to block the sodium channel.

Several studies have been performed comparing the cardiotoxic properties of ropivicaine, bupivacaine, and lidocaine (21–26). All have revealed less cardiotoxicity with ropivacainewhen compared to bupivacaine. For example, in the study by Nancarrow and colleagues, fatal doses of ropivacaine, bupivacaine, and lidocaine were established in awake sheep (24). The ratios of fatal doses found was 1:2:9 (3.7:7.3:30.8 mg/kg for bupivacaine, ropivacaine, and lidocaine, respectively). A study by Reiz and colleagues also demonstrated almost 50% less cardiotoxicity with ropivacaine than bupivacaine in a model of intracoronary injection in anesthetized, ventilated pigs (25). In this investigation, arrhythmogenicity was 2:4.5:30 mg, intracoronary, for bupivacaine, ropivacaine, and lidocaine, respectively. In another animal study by Feldman and colleagues, there were more fatal injections of local anesthetic in animals receiving bupivacaine (5/6) than ropivacaine (1/6) or lidocaine (2/6) (26).

Ropivicaine has been extensively studied clinically during single-shot nerve blocks. It appears to be equipotent to bupivacaine in this setting yet with slightly shorter duration of action (27–29). Specifically, ropivacaine has been found to be comparable to bupivacaine for upper extremity nerveblocks, including axillary nerve blocks (27, 30, 31), supraclavicular blocks (32), and interscalene blocks (33). Ropivicaine has also been used for ilioinguinal nerve (34), lumbar plexus (35), and sciatic/femoral nerve blocks (36). Ropivicaine has also been utilized for intravenous regional anestheisa (37, 38). In these investigations, one compared lidocaine 0.5% to ropivacaine 0.2% (37) and the other, lidocaine (3 mg/kg) to ropivacaine (1.2 and 1.8 mg/kg) (38). In both investigations, there were fewer central nervous system side effects and less prolonged residual sensory blockade in the patients receiving ropivacaine. At the present time, there are no case reports detailing cardiovascular collapse or death related to accidental intravenous injection of ropivacaine (39–41).

Three studies have evaluated the pharmacokinetic profile of epidural infusions of ropivacaine for 24 to 72 hours duration (42–44). All three studies have revealed an increase in total plasma ropivacaine concentration with time, yet the unbound concentration of drug remained relatively stable because of parallel increases in plasma levels of alpha-1-glycoprotein. Following 24 hours, an epidural ropivacaine infusion of 10 and 20 mg/h produces mean plasma unbound drug concentrations of 0.53 and 0.88 mg/L, respectively (42). For a 72-hour infusion of epidural ropivacaine, the maximum total ropivacaine plasma concentration varies from 1.1 to 5.2 mg/L, with a maximum unbound concentration varying from 0.015 to 0.150 mg/L (43). In a study by Burn and colleagues, 28 patients receiving epidural ropivacaine, 2 or 3 mg/mL solution at 10 cc/h, exhibited maximum ropivacaine plasma concentrations of 3.1 mg/L (total) and 0.091 mg/L (unbound) (44).

Two obstetrical studies have evaluated the relative potency of ropivacaine and bupivacaine by assessing the median effective dose (via a method of up-down sequential allocation) (45, 46). Both of these studies found a potency ratio of 0.6, suggesting that ropivacaine is less potent than bupivacaine. Incidentally, a similar potency ratio has been determined for intrathecal ropivicaine when compared to intratheceal bupivacaine (47). Despite these results, many comparative clinical studies have not yet determined any clinical difference in analgesic potency between the two drugs. One must be aware that when using ropivacaine viaepidural infusion, a more rapid segmental regression of the block may occur when compared to similar use of epidural bupivacaine (48). This suggests that epidural patient-controlled analgesic techniques using ropivacaine alone may require supplemental bolus doses of drug to maintain an adequate analgesic level.

Whether or not ropivacaine produces less motor block than bupivacaine is somewhat contentious. As of May 2001, there were 82 studies evaluating motor block with ropivacaine and bupivacaine. Only 23 (30%) demonstrated a statistically significant reduction in motor block with use of ropivacaine, when compared to bupivicaine (49).

In one study that investigated fixed-rate infusions of epidural bupivacaine versus epidural ropivacaine for knee surgery, there was less motor block in the ropivacaine group at all times (50). In contrast, another study revealed that patients with lumbar epidural catheters who received low concentrations (0.2% ropivacaine or 0.175% bupivacaine) of local anesthetic did not have significant differences in the incidence of lower limb motor blockade (51). Whiteside and colleagues revealed that in patients who underwent abdominal hysterectomy with thoracic epidural anesthesia (T-10), similar Bromage motor scores were observed with either bupivacaine or ropivacaine, yet significantly more patients receiving ropivacaine were able to ambulate postoperatively at the 22- and 24-hour marks (52). Brodner and colleagues revealed similar clinical results; i.e., motor recovery was faster in patients who received epidural ropivacaine when compared to patients who received epidural bupivacaine, as defined by the ability to ambulate postoperatively (53). The results of these investigations suggest that patients who receive ropivacaine via a thoracic epidural catheter may have an increased ability to ambulate in the immediate postoperative period when compared to patients receiving bupivacaine similarly.

Levobupivacaine

Levobupivacaine has essentially the same basic physicochemical properties as bupivacaine (Table 1–1). Thus, the minimum analgesic local anesthetic concentration of levobupivacaine delivered by an epidural infusion is the same by weight as bupivacaine. However, since levobupivacaine is supplied differently than bipivacaine (via weight of the unhydrated base), the molar concentration on a weight-per-weight basis of solution contains 13 % more levobupivacaine than bupivacaine. Hence, the potency of levobupivacaine is 0.87 times the potency of bupivacaine as assessed by the minimum analgesic local anesthetic model (54).

In early investigations it appeared that levobupivacaine possessed less cardiotoxic properties than bupivacaine (55, 56). In an isolated rabbit heart model, Mazoit and colleagues revealed less auriculoventricular block, less ventricular tachycardia, and less fibrillation/asystole in hearts administered levobupivacaine when compared to hearts administered R(+) bupivacaine or racemic bupivacaine (55).

In a study by Denson and colleagues, all animals receiving R(+) bupivacaine intravenously died (12/12) versus only 2/12 in the S(−) bupivacaine group (56). In a more recent investigation, Huang and colleagues, in a sheep model, revealed similar cardiac depression at subconvulsive doses for levo- and racemic bupivacaine, a lower total convulsive drug amount for levobupivacaine versus bupivacaine (75 versus 100 mg, respectively), and fewer deleterious arrhythmias associated with levobupivacaine versus bupivacaine at convulsive doses (57). Lastly, Chang and colleagues determined the lethal dose of levobupivacaine to be 227 mg intravenously, in awake sheep, versus a historic lethal dose of 156 mg of bupivacaine (58).

A double-blind, three-way crossover, electroencephalographic study involving healthy human volunteers and 10 minute intravenous infusions of 40 mg bupivacaine, 40 mg levobupivacaine, or placebo revealed significantly less central nervous system depression with levobupivacaine when compared to bupivacaine, both in terms of magnitude of effects and the area of the brain over which the effects were observed (59). In another human volunteer study (double-blind, crossover) investigating cardiovascular effects of intravenous infusions of levobupivacaine and bupivacaine, significantly less cardiac depression was observed with levobupivacaine as measured by stroke index, acceleration index, and ejection fraction when compared to bupivacaine (60).

In other clinical studies, levobupivacaine has been shown to have similar local anesthetic characteristics as bupivacaine when used for epidural anesthesia (61). When used for supraclavicular block, there is no significant difference regarding onset time, dermatomal spread, or duration of sensory and motor block, as well as overall success rate between levobupivacaine and bupivacaine (62). Levobupivacaine has also been shown to be safe and effective for ilioinguinal/iliohypogastric nerve block in children undergoing herniorrhaphy (63). Cardiovascular collapse did not occur in a case report describing accidental intravenous injection of levobupivacaine (64).

Cardiotoxicity: Ropivacaine Versus Levobupivacaine

Multiple studies have compared the cardiotoxic potentials of levobupivacaine and ropivacaine (65–71). Ericson and Avesson studied intravenous bolus injections of local anesthetics in the awake rat (65). They found that the depressant effects of ropivacaine on cardiac conduction were less than bupivacaine or levobupivacaine and that the incidence of arrhythmias was less with ropivacaine than bupivacaine or levobupivacaine (65). In another study involving intracoronary injections of local anesthetics in swine, Morrison and colleagues revealed that total lethal doses of levobupivacaine and ropivacaine were lower than bupivacaine and that higher doses of levobupivacaine and ropivacaine were required to induce QRS widening than bupivacaine (QRS prolongation potency ratio: 2.1:1.4:1.1 for bupivacaine, levobupivacaine, and ropivacaine, respectively) (66). Mazoit and colleagues duplicated these results in an in vitro model of isolated rabbit heart (67). In this investigation, QRS prolongation ratio was higher for bupivacaine than either levobupivacaine or ropivacaine (1:0.4:0.3 for bupivacaine, levobupivacaine, and ropivacaine, respectively). Sudo and colleagues, in an in vitro model of isolated rat ventricular muscle strips, revealed similar depression of contractility in ventricular muscle fibers exposed to both levobupivacaine or bupivacaine, yet less depression of contractility in those fibers exposed to ropivacaine when compared to the bupivacaine isomers (68).

Groban and colleagues have extensively investigated the cardiotoxic properties of the new local anesthetics (69–71). In an anesthetized/ventilated dog model, they studied the incidence of ventricular dysrhythmias with or without programmed electrical stimulation (PES) during targeted plasma concentrations of local anesthetics produced by a graded intravenous infusion. The incidence of PES-induced extrasystoles was more frequent during bupivacaine infusion and levobupiva-caine infusion when compared to similar ropivacaine or lidocaine infusions. The incidence of spontaneous or PES-induced ventricular tachy-cardia and ventricular fibrillation did not differ among the different local anesthetics studied. The lack of a reduction in premature ventric-ular contractions with levobupivacaine infusion provides evidence against stereoselective arrhythmogenesis as the primary component of local anesthetic-induced cardiotoxicity (69).

In another study by Groban and colleagues, they determined the local anesthetic plasma concentration needed to increase the left ven-tricular end-diastolic pressure by 25% and to decrease indices of my-ocardial contractility (dP/dT, ejection fraction, fractional area of short-ening, cardiac output) by 35 %. Higher ropivacaine and lidocaine plasma concentrations were required to reach these end-points when compared to levobupivacaine and bupivacaine plasma concentrations (Table 1–2) (70). These same investigators also studied resuscitability following cardiovascular collapse due to local anesthetic injection. Forty dogs received escalating intravenous infusions of ropivacaine, levobupivacaine, bupivacaine, or lidocaine (until mean arterial pres-sure < 45 mm Hg). Following administration of intravenous epineph-rine and application of the advanced cardiac life support protocol, there was a clinically significant difference in mortality between bupivicaine-and levobupivacaine-infused dogs (50% and 30%, respectively) when compared to ropivacaine- and lidocaine-infused animals (10% and 0%, respectively). The free plasma concentration of ropivacaine leading to cardiovascular collapse (median 19.8 mcg/ml, range [10, 39]) in these

TABLE 1–2. Local Anesthetic Concentration Required to Depress Cardiac Function

Local anesthetic	LVEDP (125%)	dP/dt	%EF	%FS	CO
		(65%)	(65%)	(65%)	(65%)
Bupivacaine	2.20	2.30	3.22	2.12	3.57
	(1.15–4.4)	(1.73–3.05)	(2.22–4.66)	(1.47–3.08)	(2.10–6.05)
Levobupivacaine	1.65	2.42	3.09	1.26	3.34
	(0.87–3.13)	(1.88–3.12)	(1.44–2.87)	(0.89–1.79)	(2.03–5.51)
Ropivacaine	3.98	4.03	4.25	2.95	5.04
	(2.1–7.54)*	(3.13–5.19)#	(2.99–6.04)	(2.07–4.19)*	(3.06–8.32)

Note: The data represent the estimated concentration for 50% of a population.
Units are microgram/ml.
*ropivacaine > levobupivacaine; $P < 0.05$
#ropivacaine > bupivacaine, levobupivacaine; $P < 0.05$
Source: Adapted from Reference 70.

animals was higher than bupivacaine (median 5.7 mcg/ml, range [3,11]) or levobupivacaine (median 9.4 mcg/m, range [5,18]), suggesting a greater margin of safety with ropivacaine (71).

SUSTAINED-RELEASE FORMULATION OF TRADITIONAL DRUGS

A current trend in analgesic drug development is to produce drugs that can be delivered in the epidural space that provides analgesia for extended periods of time via a controlled-release mechanism.

Liposomal Delivery Systems

Liposomes are microscopic liquid vesicles formed when dry lipids are suspended in an excessof water. The resulting vesicle structure consists of one or many aqueous compartments surrounded by one or more lipid bilayers. The lipid bilayers offer resistance to the entrapped substance; thus, the liposome functions as a vehicle to deliver drugs in high concentrations to specific targets over time while avoiding possible systemic drug toxicity because of the limited bioavailability of the drug. The size and the structure of the liposome, as well as the composition of the bilayers profoundly affect the kinetics of drug delivery (72).

Depo-Morphine

SkyePharma, Incorporated, San Diego, California, has developed a sustained-release formulation of morphine sulfate using its DepoFoam proprietary drug delivery system. DepoFoam particles are synthetic replicas of natural lipids (liposomes) and are biodegradable and biocompatible. In rats, epidural implantation of sustained-release morphine (morphine encapsulated in multivesicular liposomes) permitted the delivery of large doses of morphine into the epidural space, producing substantial analgesia for extended periods of time without increasing side effects of the drug (73). In dogs, epidurally administered sustained-release morphine demonstrated a slower time to onset of analgesia yet a much longer duration of action (62 hours) when compared to conventional epidural morphine (27 hours) (74). In human investigations, sustained-release epidural morphine at doses of 10, 20, and 30 mg, administered epidurally to 19 patients undergoing total hip arthroplasty about 1 hour before surgery, substantially improved ambulatory tolerance (ability for sustained walking on level ground) at 72 hours postoperatively (75). The greatest ambulatory tolerance was noted in patients receiving 20 mg (versus 10 and 30 mg) and significant postoperative intravenous opioid sparing effect was observed, along with improved analgesia during activity. Moreover, there was less sedation in patients receiving 20 mg when compared to patients receiving 30 mg and placebo (intravenous fentanyl, patient-controlled analgesia) (75). In a similar study presented at the 2001 American Pain Society Meeting, similar results were reported in 37 patients (between the ages of 18 and 65 years) who underwent total hip arthroplasty. In this study, patients in the placebo group required intravenous rescue fentanyl at 5.9 hours postoperatively whereas those in the treatment groups (sustained-release epidural morphine) required rescue fentanyl at the 29.6 hour mark postoperatively. Furthermore, mean total fentanyl use during the immediate postoperative period (from 0 to 48 hours) was eight times higher in the placebo group when compared to the patients receiving sustained-release epidural morphine.

The clear advantage in treating patients with sustained-release epidural morphine is that an epidural catheter is not required for the continuous delivery of epidural analgesics. Since the use of fractionated heparin has dramatically increased in these types of surgical patients, one can thus still provide them with epidural analgesics that appear to be superior to conventional intravenous patient-controlled analgesics for up to 72 hours postoperatively.

Liposomal Bupivacaine

Attempts have also been made to incorporate local anesthetics into liposomes. In a mouse model, sensory block was significantly increased (130 versus 46 minutes) with liposomal bupivacaine when compared to plain bupivacaine (76). Moreover, the bupivacaine dose that was lethal to half of the animals administered the drug was significantly higher for those animals receiving liposomal bupivacaine (291 mg/kg versus 61 mg/kg, respectively) when compared to animals receiving plain bupivacaine (76). Also, use of liposomal bupivacaine in humans for postsurgical and cancer pain has been reported (77, 78). However, liposomal bupivacaine continues to undergo development and it is not clear when it will be available for clinical use.

Bupivacaine/Polyester Microspheres

Investigators have studied the properties of microspheres prepared with polylactic-coglycolic acid polymers loaded with bupivacaine. In peripheral nerve blockade studies, 5.5 days block duration was obtained on rat sciatic nerve preparations (79). Interestingly, the addition of glucocorticoid to the microspheres prolonged the block by a magnitude of 5 to 13 (79, 80). During intercostal nerve blockade with bupivacaine microspheres in sheep, doses of 80 mg/kg (with dexamathasone) produced 13 days block duration. In this study, plasma levels of bupivacaine remained 10-fold below the known convulsive EC50 concentration for sheep. Also, chest wall histology showed substantial granulomatous reaction around the bupivacaine microspheres yet not around the bupivacaine-dexamethasone microspheres (81).

ZICONOTIDE (SNX-111)

Ziconotide is the synthetic form of the conus snail venom and is a selective N-type voltage-sensitive calcium-channel blocker. Following intrathecal administration, it produces substantial antinociception in rat models of acute, persistent, neuropathic, and postoperative pain (82–85). In humans, there are reports of clinical effectiveness in AIDS patients (86) and a case report describes successful therapy with the drug in a patient with a 23-year history of upper phantom limb pain (87). Evidence also exists that indicates the drug may be useful in controlling postoperative pain (88) and two case reports detail its use in patients with spasticity (89). However, side effects of the drug (hypotension and/or bradycardia from sympathetic blockade) can be profound (90).

The availability of a new analgesic drugs for intrathecal administration that utilize different analgesic pathways than opioids, local anesthetics, and clonidine would be a welcome addition to our armamentarium. Unfortunately, the results of initial investigations in the acute pain setting have not been very encouraging with ziconotide and it appears that its clinical applicability will be primarily in the chronic pain management area. Furthermore, it is noteworthy that phase III studies were completed on ziconotide a few years ago in a large group of patients with malignant pain and the drug is still not yet clinically available.

PERIPHERAL OPIOID RECEPTOR ANTAGONISTS

One of the common side effect of opioids is constipation. It remains a substantial problem in approximately 40% of patients receiving opioids for metastatic cancer pain and is a common postoperative problem on surgical wards (91, 92). Animal investigations reveal a constipating/analgesic dose ratio ranging from 4 to 20 for opioids (93, 94). The constipating effect of morphine is mediated by mu and delta opioid receptors. Physiologically, morphine inhibits gastric emptying, reduces intestinal secretion, increases intestinal fluid absorption, and reduces propulsive peristalsis of the intestine, hence causing constipation. Nonselective opioid receptor antagonists (naloxone, naltrexone, and nalmefene) may reduce constipation, yet these drugs all cross the blood–brain barrier and thus have the potential to reverse analgesia (95). This is the rationale (decreasing drug penetration of the blood–brain barrier) for the development of the new peripheral opioid receptor antagonists such as methylnaltrexone and ADL 8–2698.

Methylnaltrexone

Adding a methyl group to naltrexone forms a compound, methynaltrexone, with greater polarity and lower lipid solubility. Methylnaltrexone does not cross the blood–brain barrier. In an initial clinical study performed on 12 healthy human volunteers, intravenous methylnaltrexone prevented morphine-induced oral-cecal transit delay without reversing morphine-induced analgesia (96). In a subsequent controlled clinical trial, intravenous methylnaltrexone significantly improved oral-cecal transit time in human subjects on a methadone maintenance program without precipating opioid withdrawl (97). An oral form of methylnaltrexone is also under development and has the clinical potential to treat other peripherally mediated opioid side effects such as nausea and itching (98, 99).

ADL 8-2698

ADL 8-2698 is an orally active, intestinal selective, peripherally restricted, reversible, competitive opioid antagonist undergoing active development (phase II/III) by Adolor Corporation. In a phase II postoperative ileus efficacy and dose range study, 78 patients (15 partial colectomies, 36 simple hysterectomies, and 27 radical hysterectomies) were randomized to receive either placebo or ADL 8-2698 (1 mg twice per day or 6 mg twice per day). Patients receiving the 6 mg dose experienced significantly shorter time to eat a solid diet (1.3 days faster), significantly shorter time to first bowel movement (2 days faster), and significantly shorter time to hospital discharge (1 day faster) when compared to patients receiving placebo. Also, none of the patients receiving the 6 mg dose of ADL 8-2698 experienced vomiting whereas 23% in the placebo group did experience vomiting. Furthermore, ADL 8-2698 did not antagonize analgesia (100). In other clinical studies, the drug has not induced withdrawal symptoms in chronic pain patients or methadone maintenance patients and has not antagonized pupil constriction in volunteers receiving intravenous or oral morphine.

The clinical availability of a reliable peripheral opioid antagonist would have tremendous implications on the way patients recover after surgery. Moreover, the economic implications would be substantial, as patients could potentially be discharged earlier from the hospital (once they tolerate a regular diet and ambulate without pain).

SUMMARY

The most important, clinically relevant, recent advances in regional anesthesia include the development of new local anesthetics (ropivacaine, levobupivacaine) that possess less cardiotoxic properties, initiate less central nervous system depression, and are associated with less motor blockade than traditional local anesthetics (bupivacaine). Other important advances include development of sustained-release formulations of traditional drugs (morphine, local anesthetics), which may permit delivery of drugs in high concentrations to specific targets over time while avoiding possible systemic drug toxicity and development of peripheral opioid receptor antagonists that do not cross the blood–brain barrier (methylnaltrexone, ADL 8–2698), which may reduce traditional side effects of opioids without affecting quality of analgesia.

References

1. Rogers A, Walker N, Schug S, McKee A, Kehlet H, van Zundert A, Sage D, Futter M, Saville G, Clark T, MacMahon S: Reduction of postoperative mortality and morbidity with epidural or spinal anesthesia: Results from overviews of randomised trials. Br Med J 321:1–12, 2000
2. Scott DA, Beilby DSN, McClymont C: Postoperative analgesia using epidural infusions of fentanyl with bupivacaine. Anesthesiology 83:727–737, 1995
3. Liu SS, Allen HW, Olsson GL: Patient-controlled epidural analgesia with bupivacaine and fentanyl on hospital wards. Anesthesiology 88:688–685, 1998
4. de Leon-Casasola OA, Parker B, Lema MJ, Harrison P, Massey J: Postoperative epidural bupivacaine-morphine therapy. Anesthesiology 81:368–375, 1994
5. Albright GA: Cardiac arrest following regional anesthesia with etidocaine or bupivacaine. Anesthesiology 51:285–287, 1979
6. Long WB, Rosenblum S, Grady IP: Successful resuscitation of bupivacaine-induced cardiac arrest using cardiopulmonary bypass. Anesthesia Analgesia 69:403–406, 1989

7. Auroy Y, Narchi P, Messiah A, Litt L, Rouvier B, Samii K: Serious complications related to regional anesthesia. Anesthesiology 88:479–486, 1997

8. Hawkins JL, Koonin MN, Palmer SK, Gibbs CP: Anesthesia-related deaths during obstetric delivery in the United States, 1979–1990. Anesthesiology 86:277–284, 1997

9. Clarkson CW, Hondeghem LM: Mechanisms for bupivacaine depression of cardiac conduction: Fast block of sodium channels during the action potential with slow recovery from block during diastole. Anesthesiology 62:396–405, 1985

10. Valenzueal C, Snyders DJ, Bennett PB: Stereoselective block of cardiac sodium channels by bupivacaine in guinea pig ventricular myocytes. Circulation 92:3014–3024, 1995

11. Valenzuela C, Delpon E, Tamkkun: Stereoselective block of human cardiac potassium channel (Kv1.5) by bupivacaine enantiomers. Biophysic J 69:418–427, 1995

12. Coyle DE, Sperelakis N: Bupivacaine and lidocaine blockade of calcium-mediated slow action potentials in guinea pig ventricular muscle. J Pharmacol Exp Ther 242:1001–1005, 1987

13. Zapata-Sudo G, Trachez MM, Sudo RT: Is comparative cardiotoxicity of $S(-)$ and $R(+)$ bupivacaine related to enantiomer-selective inhibition of L-type $Ca2+$ channels? Anesthesia Analgesia 92:496–501, 2001

14. Butterworth JF IV, James RL, Grimes J: Structure-affinity relationships and stereospecificity of several homologous series of local anesthetics for the beta-2 adrenergic receptor. Anesthesia Analgesia 85:336–342, 1997

15. Komai H, Lokuta AJ: Interaction of bupivacaine and tetracaine with sarcoplasmic reticulum $Ca2+$ release channels of skeletal and cardiac muscles. Anesthesiology 90:835–843, 1999

16. Stark F, Malgat M, Dabadie P: Comparison of the effects of bupivacaine and ropivacaine on heart cell mitichondrial bioenergetics. Anesthesiology 88:1340–1349, 1998

17. Liu P, Feldman HS, Covino BM: Acute cardiovasuclar toxicity of intravenous amide local anesthetics in anesthetized ventilated dogs. Anesthesia Analgesia 61:317–322, 1982

18. Kotelko DM, Schneider SM, Dailey PA: Bupivacaine-induced cardiac arrhythmias in sheep. Anesthesiology 60:10–18, 1984

19. Chadwick HS: Toxic and resuscitation in lidocaine or bupivacaine-infused cats. Anesthesiology 63:385–390, 1985

20. Buffington CW: The magnitude and duration of direct myocardial depression following intracoronary local anesthetics: A comparison of lidocaine and bupivacaine.Anesthesiology 70:280–287, 1989

21. Dony P, Dewinde V, Vandrick B, et al: The comparative toxicity of ropivacaine and bupivacaine at equipotent doses in rats.. Anesthesia Analgesia 91:1489–1492, 2000

22. Santos AC, Arthur GR, Wlody D, et al: Comparative systemic toxicity of ropivacaineand bupivacaine in nonpregnant and pregnant ewes. Anesthesiology 82:732–740, 1995

23. Feldman HS, Arthur GR, Pitkanen M, et al: Treatment of acute systemic toxicity after the rapid intravenous injection of ropivacaine and bupivacaine in the conscious dog. Anesthesia Analgesia 73:373–384, 1991

24. Nancarrow C, Rutten AJ, Runciman WB, Mather LE, Carapetis RJ, McLean CF, Hipkins SF: Myocardial and cerebral drug concentrations and the mechanisms of death after fatal intravenous doses of lidocaine, bupivacaine and ropivacaine in the sheep. Anesthesia Analgesia 69:276–283, 1989

25. Reiz S, Haggmark S, Johansson G, et al.: Cardiotoxicity of ropivacaine—A new amide local anaesthetic agent. Acta Anaesthesiol Scand 33:93–98, 1989

26. Feldman HS, Arthur GR, Covino BG: Comparative systemic toxicity of convulsants and supraconvulsants doses of intravenous ropivacaine, bupivacaine and lidocaine in the conscious dog. Anesthesia Analgesia 69:794–801, 1989

27. Bertini L, Tagariello V, Mancini S, et al: 0.75% and 0.5% ropivacaine for axillary brachial block: A clinical compraison with 0.5% bupivacaine. Reg Anesth Pain Med 24:514–518, 1999

28. Whiteside J: Regional anesthesia with ropivacaine. Reg Anesth Pain Med 25:659 (letter), 2000

29. Bertini L, Benedetto BD: Equipotency of ropivacaine and bupivacaine in peripheral nerve block. Reg Anesth Pain Med 25:659–660 (letter), 2000

30. McGlade DP, Kalpokas MV, Mooney PH, et al: A comparison of 0.5% ropivacaine and 0.5% bupivacaine for axillary brachial plexus aneasthesia. Aneasth Intensive Care 26:515–520, 1998

31. Vilho V, Ermo H, Teija H, et al: A clinical and pharmacokinetic comparaison of ropivacaine and bupivacaine in axillary plexus block. Anesthesia Analgesia 81:534–538, 1995

32. Vaghadia H, Chan V, Ganapathy S, et al: A multicentre trial of ropivacaine 7.5 mg/mL vs bupivacaine 5 mg/mL for supraclavicular brachial plexus anesthesia. Can J Anesth 46:946–951, 1999

33. Klein S, Greengrass RA, Steele S, et al: A comparison of 0.5% bupivacaine and 0.75% ropivacaine for interscalene brachial plexus block. Anesthesia Analgesia 87:1316–1319, 1998

34. Wulf H, Worthman F, Behnke H, et al: Pharmacokinetics and pharmacodynamics of ropivacaine 2 mg/ml, 5 mg/ml, or 7.5 mg/mL

after ilioninguinal blockage for inguinal hernia repair in adults. Anesthesia Analgesia 89:1471–1474, 1999

35. Greengrass RA, Klein SM, D'Ercole FJ, et al: Lumbar plexus block for knee arthroplasty: Comparison of ropivacaine and bupivacaine. Can J Anesth 45:1094–1096, 1998

36. Fanelli G, Casati A, Beccaria P, et al: A double blind comparison of ropivacaine, bupivacaine and mepivacaine during sciatic and femoral nerve blockade. Anesthesia Analgesia 87:597–600, 1998

37. Hartmannsgruber MWB, Silverman DG, Halaszynski TM, Bobart V, Brull SJ, Wilkerson C, Loepke AW, Atanassoff PG: Comparison of ropivacaine 0.2% and lidocaine 0.5% for intravenous regional anesthesia in volunteers. Anesthesia Analgesia 89:727–731, 1999

38. Chan VWS, Weisbrod MJ, Kaszas Z, Dragomir C: Comparison of ropivacaine and lidocaine for intravenous regional anesthesia in volunteers. Anesthesiology 90: 1602–1608, 1999

39. Selander D, Sjovall J, Waldenlind: Accidental IV injection of ropivacaine: Clinical experiences of six cases. Reg Anesth 22:70 (abstract), 1997

40. Ala-Kokko TI, Loponen A, Alahuta S: Two instances of central nervous system toxicity in the same patient following repeated ropivacaine-induced brachial plexus block. Acata Anaesthesiol Scand 44:623–626, 2000

41. Reutsch YA, Fattinger KE, Boreat A: Ropivacaine-induced convulsions and severe cardiac dysrrhythmia after sciatic nerve block. Anesthesiology 90:1784–1786, 1999

42. Erichsen CJ, Sjovall J, Kehlet H, Hedlund C, Arvidsson: Pharmacokinetics and analgesic effect of ropivacaine during continuous epidural infusion for postoperative pain relief. Anesthesiology 84:834–842, 1996

43. Scott DA, Emanuelsson BM, Mooney PH, Cook RJ, Junestrand C: Pharmacokinetics and efficacy of long-term epidural ropivacaine infusion for post-operative analgesia. Anesthesia Analgesia 85:1322–1330, 1997

44. Burn AGL, Stienstra R, Brouwer RP, Emanuelsson BM, van Kleef JW: Epidural infusion of ropivacaine for postoperative analgesia after major orthopedic surgery. Anesthesiology 93:395–403, 2000

45. Capogna G, Celleno D, Fusco P, et al: Relative potencies of bupivacaine and ropivacaine for analgesia in labour. Br J Anaesth 82:371–373, 1999

46. Polley LS, Columb MO, Naughton NN, et al: Relative analgesic potencies of ropivacaine and bupivacaine for epidural analgesia in labor. Anesthesiology 90:944–950, 1999

47. Gautier PE, De Kock M, Van Steenberge A: Intrathecal ropivacaine for ambulatory surgery. Anesthesiology 91:1239–1245, 1999

48. Scott DA: Ropivacaine for postoperative analgesia. Tech Reg Anesth Pain Manage 5:64–69, 2001
49. de Leon-Casasola: personal communication
50. Muldoon T, Milligan K, Quinn P, et al: Comparison between extra-dural infusion of ropivacaine or bupivacaine for the prevention of postoperative pain after total knee arthroplasty. Br J Anaesth 80:680–681, 1998
51. Hodgson PS, Liu SS: A comparison of ropivacaine with fentanyl to bupivacaine with fentanyl for postoperative patient-controlled epidural analgesia. Anesthesia Analgesia 92:1024–1028, 2001
52. Whiteside R, Jones D, Bignell S, et al: Epidural ropivacaine with fentanyl following major gynaecological surgery: The effect of volume and concentration on pain relief and motor impairment. Br J Anaesth 84:720–724, 2000
53. Brodner G, Mertes N, Van Aken H, Pogatzki E, Buerkle H, Marcus MA, Mollhof T: Epidural analgesia with local anesthetics after abdominal surgery: Earlier motor recovery with 0.2% ropivacaine than 0.175% bupivacaine. Anesthesia Analgesia 88:128–133, 1999
54. Lyons, G, Columb MO, Wilson RC, et al: Epidural pain relief in labour: Potencies of levobupivacaine and racemic bipivacaine. Br J Anaesth 81: 899–901, 1998
55. Mazoit JX, Noîco O, Samii K: Myocardial uptake of bupivacaine: II. Pharmacokinetics and pharmacodynamics of bupivacaine enantiomers in the isolated perfused rabbit heart. Anesthesia Analgesia 77:477–482, 1993
56. Denson DD, Behbehani MM, Gregg RV: Enantiomer-specific effects of an intravenously administered arrhytmogenic dose of bupivacaine on neurons of the nucleus tractus solitarius and the cardiovascular system in the anesthetized rat. Regional Anesthesia 17:311–316, 1992
57. Huang YF, Pryor ME, Mather LE, Veering BT: Cardiovascular and central nervous system effects of intravenous levobupivacaine and bupivacaine in sheep. Anesthesia Analgesia 86:797–804, 1998
58. Chang DH, Ladd LA, Wilson KA, et al: Tolerability of large-dose intravenous levobupivacaine in sheep. Anesthesia Analgesia 91:671–679, 2000
59. Van F, Rolan PE, Brennan N, Gennery B: Differential effects of levo- and racemic bupivavaine on the EEG in volunteers. Reg Anaesth Pain Med 23(S):35(abstract), 1998
60. Bardsley H, Gristwood, Baker H, Watson N, Nimmo W: A comparison of the cardiovascular effects of levobupivacaine and rac-bupivacaine following intravenous administration to healthy volunteers. Br J Clin Pharmacol 46:245–249, 1998
61. Cox CR, Faccenda KA, Gilooly C, Bannister J, Scott NB, Morisson

LMM: Extradural S(−)-bupivacaine: Comparison with racemic RS-bupivacaine. Br J Anaesthesia 80:289–293, 1998

62. Cox CR, Checketts, Mackenzie N, Scott NB, Bannister J: Comparison of S(−)-bupivacaine with racemic RS-bupivacaine in supraclavicular brachial plexus block. Br J Anaesthesia 80:594–598, 1998

63. Gunter JB, Gregg TL, Wittkugel EP, Varughese AM, Berlin RE, Ness D, Overbeck D: Ilioinguinal/iliohypogastric nerve block with levobupivacaine in children. Reg Anaesth Pain Med 23(S):54(abstract), 1998

64. Kopacz DJ, Allen HW: Accidental intravenous bupivacaine. Anesthesia Analgesia 90:1784–1786, 1999

65. Ericson AC, Avesson M: Effects of ropivacaine, bupivacaine and (S)-bupivacaine on the ECG after rapid IV injections to conscious rats. Int Monitor Reg Anaesthesia 8:51(abstract), 1996

66. Morrison SG, Dominguez JJ, Frascarolo P, et al: A comparison of the electrocardio—graphic vardiotoxic effects of racemic bupivacaine, levobupivacaine, and ropivacaine in anesthetized swine. Anesthesia Analgesia 90:1308–1314, 2000

67. Mazoit JX, Descaux A, Bouaziz H, Edouard A: Comparative ventricular electrophysiologic effect of racemic bupivacaine, levobupivacaine and ropivacaine on the isolated rabbit heart. Anesthesiology 93:784–792, 2000

68. Sudo RT, Trachez MM, Zapata-Sudo G: Comparative cardiac effects of R(+) and S(−) bupivacaine with ropivacaine. Anesthesiology 93:A131 (abstract), 2000

69. Groban L, Deal DD, Vernon JS, James RL, Butterworth J: Ventricular arrhythmias with or without programmed electrical stimulation after incremental overdosage with lidocaine, bupivacaine, levobupivacaine, and ropivacaine. Anesthesia Analgesia 91:1103–1111, 2000

70. Groban L, Deal DD, Vernon JC et al: Local anesthetic stereoselectivity and structure predict myocardial depression in anesthetized canines. Presented at the International Society of Regional Anesthesiologists Congress, Québec, Canada, May 31th to June 3rd, 2000 (abstract)

71. Groban L, Deal DD, Vernon JC, et al: Resuscitation after incremental overdosage withlidocaine, bupivacaine, levobupivacaine, and ropivacaine in anesthetized dogs. Anesthesia Analgesia 92:37–43, 2001

72. Grant GJ, Bansinath M: Liposomal delivry systems for local anesthetics. Reg Anesth Pain Med 26:61–63, 2001

73. Kim T, Murdande S, Gruber A, Kim S: Sustained-release morphine for epidural analgesia in rats. Anesthesiology 85:331–338, 1996

74. Yaksh TL, Provencher JC, Rathbun ML, Kohn FR: Pharmacokinetics and efficacy of epidurally delivered sustained-release encapsulated morphine in dogs. Anesthesiology90:1402–1412, 1999

75. Hartrick CT, Greene P, Kovan J: Preoperative sustained-release epidural morphine improves discharge ambulatory tolerance following total hip arthroplasty. Reg Anesth Pain Med 26(S):33 (abstract), 2001.

76. Grant GJ, Vermeulen K, Langerman L, Zakowski M, Turndorf H: Prolonged analgesia with liposomal bupivacaine in a mouse model. Regional Anesthesia 19:264–269, 1994

77. Boogaerts JG, Lafont ND, Declercq AG, Luo HC, Gravet ET, Blanchi JA, Legros FJ: Epidural administration of liposome-associated bupivacaine for the management of postsurgical pain: A first study. J Clin Anesthesia 6:315–320, 1994.

78. Lafont ND, Legros FJ, Boogaerts JG: Use of liposome-associated bupivacaine in a cancer pain syndrome. Anaesthesia 51:578–579, 1996

79. Curley J, Casstillo J, Hotz J, Uezona M, Hernandez S, Lin JO, Tigner J, Chasin M, Langer R, Berde C: Prolonged regional nerve blockade. Anesthesiology 84: 1401–1410, 1996

80. Castillo J, Curley J, Hotz, Uezono M, Tigner J, Chasin M, Wilder R, Langer R, Berde C: Glucocorticoids prolong rat sciatic nerve blockade in vivo from bupivacaine microspheres. Anesthesiology 85:1157–1166, 1996

81. Drager C, Benziger D, Gao F, Berde CB: Prolonged intercostal nerve blockade in sheep using controlled-release of bupivacaine and dexamethasone from polymer microspheres. Anesthesiology 89:969–979, 1998

82. Wang YX, Gao D, Pettus M, Phillips C, Bowersox SS: Interactions of intrathecally ziconotide, a selective blocker of neuronal N-type voltage-sensitive calcium channels, with morphine on nociception in rats. Pain 84:271–281, 2000

83. Malmberg AB, Yaksh TL: Effects of continuous intrathecal infusion of w-conopeptides, N-type calcium-channel blockers, on behavior and antinociception in the formalin and hot-plate tests in rats. Pain 60:83–90, 1995

84. Bowersoc SS, Gadbois T, Singh T, Pettus M, Wang YX, Luther RR: Selective N-type neuronal voltage sensitive calcium channel blocker, SNX-111, produces spinal antinociception in rat model of acute, persistent and neuropathic pain. J Pharmacol Exp Ther 279:1243–1249, 1996

85. Wang XY, Pettus M, Gao D, Phillips C, Bowersox SS: Effects of intrathecal administration of ziconotide, a selective neuronal N-type calcium channel blocker, on mechanical allodynia and heat hyperalgesia in a rat model of postoperative pain. Pain 84:151–158, 2000

86. Brose M, Pfeiffer WG, Hassenbusch BL, Burchiel SJ, Byas-Smith KJ, Krames E, McGuire D, Tich N, Luther RR: Analgesia produced by SNX-111 in patients with morphine-resistant pain. Proceedings

of the 15th annual scientific meeting of the American Pain Society 1996: A122(abstract).

87. Brose WG, Gutlove DP, Luther RR, Bowersox SS, McGuire D: Use of intrathecal SNX-111, a novel, N-type, voltage-sensitive, calcium channel blocker, in the management of intractable brachial plexus avulsion pain. Clin J Pain13:256–259, 1997

88. Atanassoff PG, Hartmannsgruber MW, Trasher J, Wermeling D, Longton W, Gaeta R, Singh T, Mayo M, McGuire D, Luther RR: Ziconotide, a new N-type calcium channel blocker, administered intrathecally for acute post-operative pain. Reg Anesth Pain Med25:274–278, 2000

89. Ridgeway B, Wallace M, Gerayli A: Ziconotide for the treatment of severe spasticity after spinal cord injury. Pain 85:287–289, 2000

90. Penn RD, Paice JA: Adverse effects associated with the intrathecal administration of ziconotide. Pain 85:291–296, 2000

91. Walsh TD: Oral morphine in chronic cancer pain. Pain 18:1–11, 1984

92. Glare P, Lickiss JP: Unrecognized constipation in patients with advanced cancer: A recipe for therapeutic disaster. J Pain Symp Manage 7:369–371, 1992

93. Green AF: Comparative effects of analgesics on pain threshold, respiratory frequency and gastrointestinal propulsion. Br J Pharmacol 14:26–34, 1959

94. Niemegeers C, Lenearts F, Awouters F: Preclinical animal studies of modern antidiarrheal: In vivo pharmacology. In: Van Bever W, Lal H, eds: Synthetic antidiarrheal drugs: Synthesis-preclinical and clinical pharmacology. New York, NY: Dekker, 1976:65–114

95. Sikes NP: Oral naloxone in opioids-associated constipation. Lancet 337:1475, 1991

96. Yuan CS, Foss JF, O'Connor M, Toledano A, Roizen MF, Moss J: Methylnaltrexone prevents morphine-induced delay in oral-cecal transit time without affecting analgesia: A double-blind randomized placebo-controlled trial. Clin Pharmacol Ther 59:469–475, 1996

97. Yuan CS, Foss JF, O,Connor M, Osinski J, Karrison T, Moss J, Roizen MF: Methylnaltrexone for reversal of constipation due to chronic methadome use. JAMA283:367–372, 2000

98. Yuan CS, Foss JF, Osinski J, Toledano A, Roizen MF, Moss J: The safety and efficacy of oral methylnaltrexone in preventing morhine-induced delay in oral-cecal transit time. Clin Pharmacol Ther 61:467–475, 1997

99. Yuan CS, Foss JF, Osinski J, Roizen MF, Moss J: Efficacy of orally administered methylnaltrexone in decreasing subjective effects after intravenous morphine. Drug Alcohol Dependence 52:161–165, 1998

100. Data on file, Adolor Corporation

Norbert Rolf, M.D., Ph.D.

2 | Thoracic Epidural Anesthesia in Cardiac Risk Patients

PHYSIOLOGY AND PATHOPHYSIOLOGY

In a resting adult of 70 kg body weight, coronary blood flow (CBF) is approximately 225 ml/min^{-1}, which is about 4% to 5% of cardiac output. In the autoregulatory range, CBF is nearly constant over a wide range of perfusion pressures. At a constant myocardial oxygen consumption, a decrease in coronary perfusion pressure causes autoregulatory vasodilation, adjusting coronary vascular resistance to maintain constant myocardial perfusion. The major variables influencing coronary flow are perfusion pressure, myocardial systolic compression, metabolic control, and neurohumoral factors. Beyond the autoregulatory range, coronary perfusion is proportionally related to coronary perfusion pressure and inversely dependent on coronary vascular resistance. Under these circumstances, changes in mean arterial pressure (MAP) are usually followed by a proportional change in CBF. Coronary perfusion pressure is commonly defined as the difference between MAP and left ventricular end-diastolic pressure. Because nearly 70% of CBF occurs during diastole and increases in heart rate are accompanied by a shortening of the duration of diastole, heart rate is also an important determinant of CBF.

Neural effects on cardiac performance and rhythm are mediated via α- and β-adrenergic receptors. Sympathetic α-adrenergic stimulation leads to a vasoconstrictive influence on epicardial vessels, where α-receptors dominate. Moreover, this vasoconstrictive activity limits va-

Regional Anesthesia for Cardiothoracic Surgery, edited by Mark Chaney,
Lippincott Williams & Wilkins, Baltimore © 2002.

sodilation in the subepicardial vessels and prevents epicardial steal. In healthy subjects, this stimulation does not necessarily lead to an increase in coronary vascular resistance as metabolic counter-regulation may mobilize substantial vasodilatory reserve, especially in the subendocardial tissue (1).

Intramyocardial and subendocardial coronary arteries are dominated by β_1-adrenergic receptors (2). The effect of β-adrenergic stimulation of coronary vessels is not clearly defined as multiple effects are mediated by β-receptors in vivo. β-stimulation causes positive inotropy and chronotropy leading to increased myocardial metabolism and oxygen consumption. Because perfusion and contraction are coupled, an increased myocardial metabolism is followed by an increase in CBF via metabolic regulation. The exact mechanism of metabolic regulation remains controversial; ATP-sensitive K^+-channel openers, adenosine, prostaglandins, neuropeptides and nitric oxide are involved. Counteracting the stimulation of β-receptors by β-blockers in resting dogs, however, resulted in a decreased CBF while the oxygen delivery/oxygen consumption ratio remained constant. Decreased CBF might be the result of reduced myocardial oxygen consumption (3).

The effects of sympathetic stimulation in patients with coronary artery disease differ from those in healthy subjects. Nabel et al. have demonstrated a constriction of atherosclerotic arteries induced by the cold pressor test, while smooth segments dilated (4) (Figure 2–1). This effect of sympathetic activation is in concordance with the finding in patients with classic angina that the diameter of the atherosclerotic artery decreased during exercise (5). Activation of sympathetic influences also has the potential to override local metabolic vasodilation, which has been shown for adenosine-infusion (6) or stress, induced

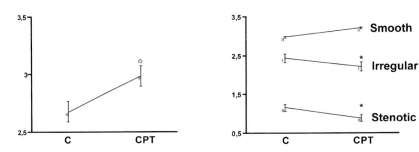

FIGURE 2–1. Effect of sympathetic stimulation by the cold pressor test (CPT) in normal volunteers (left panel) and in patients with coronary artery disease (right panel). In normal subjects, CPT leads to coronary vasodilation as compared to the control condition (C). Coronary arteries with smooth vascular wall as assessed by angiography also dilate. Vessels with irregular wall structure or with stenoses show paradoxical vasoconstriction in response to sympathetic stimulation (4).

by the cold pressor test(7). This might be caused by activation of α-receptors (8), restricting the metabolically related flow increase by about 30% (9)

Besides sympathetic reflexes, the endothelium plays an important role in the tone of coronary arteries (10). In animal studies it has been demonstrated that after removal of the endothelium, the relaxing effects of β-adrenergic agonists are reduced and the constrictive effects of α-adrenergic agonists are enhanced (11, 12). Therefore, a malfunction of the endothelium can have further deleterious effects in the mediation of sympathetic activity.

High thoracic epidural anesthesia (TEA) has the potential for blocking cardiac afferent and efferent fibers, which originate from the first to fifth thoracic level (Th_1-Th_5) (13). The perception of cardiac pain and angina is mediated via sympathetic afferent nerves. Stimulation of sympathetic efferents leads to an increase of inotropy, cardiac output, and systemic vascular resistance. Epidurally applied anesthetics targeted to the Th1-Th5 segments produce sensory blockade, motor blockade (depending on concentration), and blockade of the cardiac sympathetic fibers. In patients with coronary artery disease, it has been reported that TEA leads to a reduction in heart rate, cardiac output, and systemic vascular resistance, and it may therefore decrease myocardial oxygen demand (14, 15). However, others reported increased heart rates with reduced cardiac output (16) or no change in either value (17, 18). The effect of TEA on left ventricular contractility has been the subject of several animal and clinical studies, but it still remains controversial. Contractility has been reported to be unchanged (19, 20),reduced , (21–23), or improved (24, 25). The variability of these results might be due to different types of anesthetics used, whether or not epinephrine was added, the differing number of segments blocked and species differences. Various parameters have been used to measure left ventricular function, including isovolumetric and ejection phase indices like dP/dtmax, stroke volume, systolic time intervals or ejection fractions. All these parameters are highly dependent on cardiac loading conditions (26).

In conclusion, positive effects of TEA cannot simply be deduced from these investigations and differences in patient populations have to be taken in account when evaluating studies of TEA. Ideally, in patients at risk of ischemia, TEA should dilate constricted coronary vessels, decrease heart rate and myocardial metabolism,and improve cardiac function by reducing pre- and afterload and optimizing oxygen availability. In general, hemodynamic stability and a reduced stress response should provide an improved outcome, although hypotension can occur after epidural blockade of Th1-S5 segments by diminishing sympathetic counter-regulation in a substantial vascular reservoir (27), which may offset the positive hemodynamic effects of TEA.

EPIDURAL ANESTHESIA AND THE PATHOLOGIC STATES OF THE HEART

It has been clearly established that activation of the sympathetic nervous system plays an important role in the pathophysiology of myocardial infarction, angina pectoris, and fatal cardiac arrhythmias (28–30). Conversely, inhibition of sympathetic stimulation can reduce cardiac morbidity (31, 32). Selective inhibition of the sympathetic nervous outflow to the heart can be achived by TEA, blocking the segments Th1 to Th5, and while oxygen supply to the ischemic myocardium is improved, total CBF is unaltered. In experimental settings, the ratio of endocardial to epicardial blood flow is increased (20, 33) and blood flow to ischemic regions improved (33). Under the influence of TEA, the size of the infarcted area was smaller both in subepicardial and subendocardial regions after experimental coronary occlusion in dogs (Figure 2–2) (21, 34). After myocardial stunning, recovery was significantly faster in dogs, when the ischemic insult leading to stunning was induced during TEA under equivalent hemodynamic parameters (Figure 2–3) (20).

In humans, improvement in myocardial oxygen supply by TEA may be due to the fact that approximately 75% of coronary stenoses are dynamic and can be modulated by pharmacologic or hemodynamic

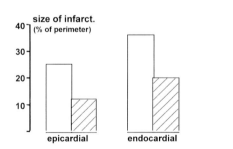
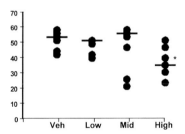

FIGURE 2–2. Effect of TEA on experimental myocardial infarction in dogs: Left panel: The percentage of the cardiac circumference occupied by infarction in 7 dogs after left anterior descending artery (LAD) occlusion. A significant decrease of the infarcted area was found in both epicardial and endocardial regions during thoracic epidural anesthesia (TEA) (modified after (21)). Right panel: Ratio of area of necrosis (AN) to area at risk (AAR). Circles represent individual animals and bars are the median for each group. VEH: vehicle group; LOW: low-dose bupivacaine in TEA (0.3 mg/kg bolus and 0.15 mg/kh/h); MID: mid-dose (0.6 mg/kg bolus and 0.3 mg/kg/h); HIGH: high-dose (1.2 mg/kg bolus and 0.6 mg/kh/h) (modified after (34)).

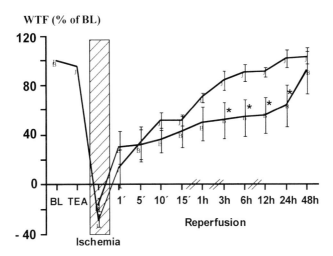

FIGURE 2–3.   Recovery of wall thickening fraction (WTF) from myocardial stunning in conscious dogs with and without thoracic epidural anesthesia (TEA). During the 48 hours reperfusion period after a 10 minute occlusion of the left anterior descending artery, dogs recovered significantly faster with TEA (modified after (20)).

interventions. By inducing a high level TEA (Th1-Th6) with bupivacaine, Blomberg et al. (24) were able to increase the luminal diameter of stenotic coronary arteries in 64% of the patients, whereas no effects were seen on nonstenotic segments. Studies have suggested that β-blockers cause a direct constriction of coronary arteries by unmasking the effect of postjunctional α-receptors. As nearly all patients in the study of Blomberg et al. (24) received β-blocker-therapy, a decrease in the stimulation of α-adrenergic receptors may have increased blood flow through arterioles with diseased endothelium. Another indicator that increased blood flow is the main determinant in improving the ratio of oxygen supply and demand during TEA is the observation that in patients with unstable angina pectoris, high level TEA reduced ST-depression at a comparable workload during an exercise stress test (35). In patients with stable angina pectoris, TEA reduced ST-depression during exercise (25, 35), although the 15% higher ejection fraction (EF) with TEA could not be explained entirely by lower RPP (25). In addition, TEA has been used to treat anginal pain after multiple attempts to stop nitrate infusion had failed (35) and for long-term treatment of anginal pain (36).

Further support that the beneficial effects of TEA are not confined to hemodynamic changes is given by an experimental study by Tsuchida et al. (27). Brief coronary occlusions (5 min) lead to ST-segment elevation and a concomitant decrease in pH, which was attenuated under TEA. This beneficial effect was also present when TEA-induced hemodynamic changes were corrected by blood transfusion or pacing. Intramyocardial levels of adenosine triphosphate (ATP), creatine phosphate, and lactate remained unchanged.

Intramyocardial energy utilization is affected by cardiac rhythm and the autonomic nervous system plays a critical role in its modulation. Several findings predict that TEA should protect against ventricular tachydysrhythmias and reentry supraventricular tachycardias but may cause atrioventricular block (38, 39). In halothane-anesthetized dogs, the dose of exogenous epinephrine required to induce arrhythmia was significantly higher with TEA using mepivacaine (40). As this effect was not seen with intravenous mepivacaine, the elevation of the arrhythmogenic threshold is not an effect of systemically absorbed local anesthetic and therefore represents an effect of sympathetic blockade by epidural anesthesia. This result is in agreement with an earlier study in rats in which the incidence of ventricular arrhythmias after coronary ligation with and without TEA was compared (41). The incidence of ventricular flutter occuring in the first 30 minutes after ligation of the left coronary artery was 53% in the control group compared with 20% in the TEA group. In awake chronically instrumented dogs, TEA increased the duration of monophasic action potentials and prolonged the effective refractory period at higher pacing rates (42).

Hypercoagulability manifested by increases in fibrinogen, platelet activity and plasminogen activator inhibitor-1 (PAI-1), commonly occurs after major surgery. It has also been implicated in the genesis of unstable angina and myocardial infarction (43). Beneficial effects of epidural anesthesia on coagulation status have been described (43, 44). The majority of studies adressing this issue used lumbar epidural anesthesia (LEA), not TEA. The Perioperative Ischemia Randomized Anesthesia Trial study group (PIRAT) (45) reported a significantly reduced rate of graft occlusions in patients undergoing lower extremity revascularization who received epidural versus general anesthesia. In patients with general anesthesia, PAI-1-activity was higher 24 hours after the operation as compared with patients who received epidural anesthesia (43). In patients undergoing major vascular surgery, Tuman et al. found only 1 thrombosis in a patient after regional anesthesia versus 11 in the general anesthesia group (46). In the epidural group, platelet aggregation was reduced postoperatively.

Beneficial effects of TEA can be caused by systemic absorption of local anesthetic leading to plasma concentrations efficient enough to directly impair platelet aggregation (47, 48). On the other hand, reduction of stress response with epidural anesthesia and analgesia may indirectly affect platelet function (49) and attenuate the catabolism of proteins involved in coagulation (46). In addition, blood inflow and venous emptying is improved (50).

LUMBAR OR THORACIC APPROACH?

An important question is whether beneficial effects can be achieved by a LEA instead of TEA. Sympathetic block leads to numerous effects on the vascular bed. Measurement of sympathetic impulses in postganglionic fibers to skin and muscle of the legs have shown a complete block of either spontaneous or induced sympathetic activity during epidural anesthesia (51). Epidural blockade of lumbar segments resulted in an increased sympathetic activity in splanchnic nerves due to baroreceptor drive, but only TEA produces near total ablation of splanchnic activity (52, 53).

However, both techniques have an inherent risk of cardiovascular depression and hypotension. The most frequent cardiovascular complications, e.g., vasovagal syncope and arterial vasodilation, are usually treated successfully with atropine and intravenous volume replacement, as well as vasopressor drugs when indicated.

Bradycardia due to the Bezold-Jarisch reflex is commonly refractory to atropine treatment and the administration of potent vasopressors. These patients experience hypotension and profound bradycardia, associated with venous blood pooling and heightened cardiac contractility (54). This results in reflex arterial dilation and vagally mediated bradycardia. Owing to the extent of the sympathetic block and vasodilation, this reflex occurs more often with LEA than with TEA.

In an experimental setting in swine, the injection of bupivacaine for LEA with blockade to the thoracic level induced a severe reduction of myocardial blood flow distal to a coronary artery stenosis (55). The reduction in oxygen supply due to hypotension during LEA is not followed by a concomitant reduction in demand (15). This might even be aggravated by an enhanced sympathetic reactivity in sympathetically intact areas (56–58), which has been demonstrated for LEA and TEA in cats (59). During TEA the lower CBF seems to be compensated by a decrease in myocardial oxygen demand and cardiac work (15). Similar reductions in mean arterial pressure are not followed by segmental wall motion disturbances during TEA (15), but they are during LEA (60). Kock et al. found an improved cardiac performance during exercise under TEA than during control exercise (25). Ischemia-induced left ventricular global and regional wall motion abnormalities was improved under TEA, associated with less pronounced ST-segment depression. In a meta-analysis of the effects of regional anesthesia on mortality, a significant reduction of mortality was demonstrated for TEA but not for

LEA (61). In conclusion, TEA has more favorable effects than LEA in the patient with coronary artery disease.

EPIDURAL ANESTHESIA IN NONCARDIAC SURGERY

As described above, TEA has been shown to have several benefits in myocardial ischemia: anginal pain is improved even when other therapies failed, the stress response to surgery is suppressed, and the incidences of myocardial infarctions and arrhythmias may be reduced. Unfortunately, there have been few studies focusing on the effect of TEA in noncardiac surgery. Thus, an evaluation needs to consider epidural anesthesia in general.

An often-quoted study has been published by Yeager et al. in 1987 (62). Even though the study can be criticized because of methodological drawbacks, its surprising results sparked further investigations. Fifty patients undergoing thoracic, abdominal, or vascular surgery were randomized into two groups. The first group received a combined anesthesia with epidural and balanced general anesthesia, the second received general anesthesia alone. The number of severe cardiovascular complications was significantly higher in the group with balanced general anesthesia alone. Four deaths occurred in this group more than 2 weeks postoperatively, while all patients in the combined anesthesia group survived. Three myocardial infarctions occurred in the general anesthesia group versus none in the combined anesthesia group.

The level of epidural anesthesia (lumbar or thoracic) was not controlled and neither were the techniques of general anesthesia nor the postoperative pain therapy standardized or specified. The study population was heterogeneous with respect to severity and invasiveness of surgery, and patients were not stratified according to concomitant diseases. The high incidence of severe complications and high mortality cast doubt on the validity of this study.

The results obtained by Yeager were not confirmed in a better-designed study by Baron et al. (63) of 173 patients undergoing aortic reconstruction. The patients were randomized in two groups receiving either a "balanced" general anesthesia or TEA in combination with light general anesthesia. Ejection fraction, associated coronary artery disease, hemodynamic parameters, and cardiovascular treatment were equally distributed in both groups. All patients received a thoracic epidural catheter, which was not used intraoperatively in the general anesthesia group. There was no difference between both groups concerning cardiovascular complications, infections, and mortality. Postoperative pain therapy, unfortunately, was not controlled or randomized, therefore no conclusions regarding the perioperative period in general can be based on this study.

The effects of epidural anesthesia during the postoperative period were investigated in a study by Tuman and coworkers (46). They randomized 80 patients suffering from atherosclerosis and undergoing major vascular surgery to compare the effects of general anesthesia (GEN) with on-demand narcotic analgesia or general anesthesia combined with epidural anesthesia and analgesia (GEN-EPI). Patients in the GEN-EPI group had high lumbar or low thoracic (L3-Th10) epidural catheters. The concomitant diseases were comparable in both groups, besides a significantly higher rate of diabetes mellitus and previous myocardial infarction in the GEN-EPI group. The rates of cardiovascular, infectious, and overall postoperative complications as well as the duration of the intensive-care-unit stay were significantly reduced in the GEN-EPI group.

A combined use of epidural and general anesthesia or general anesthesia alone during the intra- and postoperative period was performed by the PIRAT group (45) in patients with lower extremity surgery. LEA-catheters were inserted at L2-L3 or L3-L4. No differences were discovered with regard to cardiac outcomes, renal or pulmonary complications. However, the need for reoperation was reduced in the epidural group.

A more recent study by Bode et al. (64) was unable to find a statistically significant difference in the effects of lumbar regional (epidural or spinal) versus general anesthesia on perioperative cardiac morbidity and overall mortality in patients undergoing peripheral vascular surgery. Although this study is a little out of the context of this review, it is included as it provided an interesting finding: the cardiac death rate associated with an inadequate regional anesthesia necessitating conversion to a general anesthetic was significantly higher compared with that of patients having a successful regional or general anesthetic.

Recovery from epidural anesthesia is of clinical importance. Sprung et al. (65) reported two patients who developed cardiac arrest caused by coronary spasm during recovery from epidural anesthesia. They concluded that this might be caused by imbalances between parasympathetic and sympathetic nervous systems. While current data do not definitively establish the benefit of intraoperative LEA, it is clear that additional investigation is required to clarify the role of epidural analgesia postoperatively, especially when administered via the thoracic spinal segments.

TEA AND LUNG FUNCTION

As reduction of myocardial oxygen supply might be exacerbated by hypoxemia, the effect of TEA on lung function must be considered.

Impaired ventilatory function as reflected by reduced vital capacity occurs after abdominal as well as after thoracic surgery (66–69). Periods of hypoxemia occur postoperatively, especially during sleep (70–72) and are associated with myocardial ischemia (70). Impairment of lung function starts with induction of general anesthesia and lasts for 1 up to 2 weeks postoperatively.

An important approach in reducing postoperative pulmonary dysfunction is the improvement of analgesia by epidural application of local anesthetics or opioids. For opioids, the epidural route provides better recovery of pulmonary function compared with intravenous administration (73, 74). Periods of oxygen desaturation are reduced during epidural as compared with intravenous anesthesia (72).

However, pain does not seem to be the only determinant of ventilatory deterioration postoperatively. The inhibiton of diaphragmatic function despite profound analgesia plays an important role in ventilatory impairment (75–77). The precise mechanism of diaphragmatic dysfunction is unknown; one hypothesis suggests that stimulation of afferent nerves in the chest and abdominal walls, viscera, and the diaphragm leads to an inhibition of phrenic motor drive (66). TEA has been shown to improve postoperative diaphragmatic function in lambs (78) and humans 79), and to improve respiratory function parameters (80).

In contrast to these beneficial effects, TEA has potentially negative effects by paralysis of the thoracic muscles (78). The denervation of the musculature of the rib cage theoretically alters lung volumes. Measurements of functional residual capacity (FRC) before and after induction of TEA in subjects without lung disease did not reveal any changes in this muscle-tone-dependent lung volume (81). In elderly patients, Sakura et al. found a significant decrease of 13% in minute ventilation and a 14% decrease in tidal volume after induction of TEA, but no impairment in the response to hypercapnia or hypoxia (82). When LEA is extended to high thoracic levels (Th1), FRC is significantly increased (83) and associated with a reduction in intrathoracic blood volume after peripheral vasodilation. As with effects on cardiac function, the number of segments blocked seems to play an important role in the effects of TEA on lung function.

The pulmonary vasculature is innervated by the autonomic nervous system, and hypoxic pulmonary vasoconstriction may be influenced by sympathetic neural blockade. Hypoxic pulmonary vasoconstriction, an important mechanism for maintenance of adequate oxygenation after induction of general anesthesia (84), is not affected by TEA in dogs (85).

In clinical studies, a positive effect of TEA during anesthesia is mainly present in patients at high risk of postoperative pulmonary complications, but may also be observed when adequate epidural analgesia is maintained into the postoperative period (86). An important issue is the control of dynamic pain, i.e., adequate analgesia during movement in contrast to analgesia only at rest. This is important for pulmonary function, and in patients receiving epidural versus intravenous PCA treatment, pulmonary function was significantly improved. Current data do suggest that TEA reduces postoperative pulmonary complications. Reducing hypoxemic episodes in the postoperative period may help to reduce the incidence of myocardial ischemia in high risk patients.

CONCLUSIONS

Earlier editorial comments about the optimal anesthetic regimen for peripheral vascular surgery stated that the question of the "best anesthetic management for this group of these seriously ill patients" remains unresolved (87); last year it was concluded that further studies were unlikely to be useful (88). However, these editorials were based on studies that had some limitations: the use of LEA and/or the absence of postoperative epidural analgesia. A number of studies are, however, now available that support the use and initiation of further studies of TEA in patients with compromised cardiac function to obtain an answer to this important question.

TEA improves cardiac performance and may even have beneficial effects on the oxygen delivery/demand ratio. TEA has beneficial effects on several parameters (catecholamines, nitrogen balance, coagulation) that correlate with improved patient outcome, although definite proof for better outcome has not been documented. Lung function may also benefit from TEA. Outcome benefit from TEA can be reasonably expected only when its intraoperative use is extended to the postoperative period. Considering the level and extent of epidural anesthesia, data indicate that TEA is superior to LEA in patients with compromised cardiac function.

Questions still unanswered include the application of TEA in anticoagulated patients. Based upon current knowledge, application of TEA in the face of anticoagulation should be undertaken with caution and with consideration of the caveats outlined above. The optimal duration and analgesic regimen of TEA in the postoperative period also remains undefined. Finally, the optimal combination of general anesthesia (inhalational/intravenous) with intraoperative regional anesthesia has yet to be established.

References

1. Mudge GH, Grossmann W, Mills RM, Lesch M, Braunwald E: Reflex increase in coronary vascular resistance in patients with ischemic heart disease. N Engl J Med 24:1333–1337, 1976

2. Feigl EO: Coronary physiology. Physiol Rev 63:1–205, 1983
3. Heyndrickx GR, Pannier JL, Muylaert P: Alteration in myocardial oxygen balance during exercise after β-adrenergic blockade in dogs. J Appl Physiol 49:28–33, 1980
4. Nabel EG, Ganz P, Gordon JB, Alexander RW, Selwyn AP: Dilation of normal and constriction of atherosclerotic coronary arteries caused by the cold pressor test. Circulation 77:43–52, 1988
5. Gage JE, Hess OM, Murakami T, Ritter M, Grimm J, Krayenbuehl HP: Vasoconstriction of stenotic coronary arteries during dynamic exercise in patients with classic angina pectoris: reversibility by nitroglycerin. Circulation 73:865–876, 1986
6. Johannsen UJ, Mark AL, Marcus ML: Responsiveness to cardiac sympathetic nerve stimulation during maximal coronary dilation produced by adenosine. Circ Res 50:510–517, 1982
7. Mudge GH, Jr., Goldberg S, Gunther S, Mann T, Grossman W: Comparison of metabolic and vasoconstrictor stimuli on coronary vascular resistance in man. Circulation 59:544–550, 1979
8. Heusch G, Deussen A: The effects of cardiac sympathetic nerve stimulation on perfusion of stenotic coronary arteries in the dog. Circ Res 53:8–15, 1983
9. Mohrman DE, Feigl EO: Competition between sympathetic vasoconstriction and metabolic vasodilation in the canine coronary circulation. Circ Res 42:79–86, 1978
10. Furchgott RF, Jothianandan D: Endothelium-dependent and -independent vasodilation involving cyclic GMP. Blood Vessels 28:52–61, 1991
11. Miller VM, Vanhoutte PM: Muscular and endothelial responsiveness to alpha-adrenergic activation in canine bloodvessels. The Physiologist 27:282–286, 1984
12. Rubanyi GM, Vanhoutte PM: Endothelium removal decreases relaxation of coronary arteries caused by beta-adrenergic agonists and adenosine. J Cardiovasc Pharmacol 7:139–144, 1985
13. Cousins M, Bromage P: Epidural Neural Blockade.In: Cousins M, Bridenbaugh P (eds):Neural Blockade. Philadelphia: JB Lippincott, 1980:253–360
14. Blomberg S, Emanuelsson H, Ricksten SE: Thoracic epidural anesthesia and central hemodynamics in patients with unstable angina pectoris. Anesth Analg 69:558–562, 1989
15. Saada M, Catoire P, Bonnet F, Delaunay L, Gormezano G, Macquin Mavier I, Brun P: Effect of thoracic epidural anesthesia combined with general anesthesia on segmental wall motion assessed by transesophageal echocardiography. Anesth Analg 75:329–335, 1992
16. Reiz S, Nath S, Ponten E: Hemodynamic effects of prenalterol, a beta1-adrenoreceptor agonist, in hypotension induced by high

thoracic epidural block in man. Acta Anaesthesiol Scand 23:93–96, 1979

17. Sjögren S, Wright B: Circulatory changes during continuous epidural blockade. Acta Anaesthesiol Scand (Suppl) 46:5–25, 1972
18. Hasenbos M, Liem TH, Kerkkamp H, Gielen M: The influence of high thoracic epidural analgesia on the cardiovascular system. Acta Anaesthesiol Belg 39:49–54, 1988
19. Ottesen S, Renck H, Jynge P: Cardiovascular effects of epidural analgesia. I. Thoracic epidural analgesia. An experimental study in sheep of the effects on central circulation, regional perfusion and myocardial performance during normoxia, hypoxia and isoproterenol administration. Acta Anaesthesiol Scand (Suppl) 69:1–16, 1978
20. Rolf N, Van de Velde M, Wouters PF, Möllhoff T, Weber TP, Van Aken HK: Thoracic epidural anesthesia improves functional recovery from myocardial stunning in conscious dogs. Anesth Analg 83:935–940, 1996
21. Davis RF, Deboer LW, Maroko PR: Thoracic epidural anesthesia reduces myocardial infarct size after coronary artery occlusion in dogs. Anesth Analg 65:711–717, 1986
22. Hotvedt R, Platou ES, Refsum H: Effects of thoracic epidural analgesia on cardiovascular function and plasma concentration of free fatty acids and catecholamines in the dog. Acta Anaesthesiol Scand 28:132–137, 1984
23. Lundberg J, Norgren L, Thomson D, Werner O: Hemodynamic effects of dopamine during thoracic epidural anesthesia in man. Anesthesiology 66:641–646, 1987
24. Blomberg S, Emanuelsson H, Kvist H, Lamm C, Ponten J, Waagstein F, Ricksten SE: Effects of thoracic epidural anesthesia on coronary arteries and arterioles in patients with coronary artery disease. Anesthesiology 73:840–847, 1990
25. Kock M, Blomberg S, Emanuelsson H, Lomsky M, Stromblad SO, Ricksten SE: Thoracic epidural anesthesia improves global and regional left ventricular function during stress-induced myocardial ischemia in patients with coronary artery disease. Anesth Analg 71:625–630, 1990
26. Robotham JL, Takata M, Berman M, Harasawa Y: Ejection fraction revisited. Anesthesiology 74:172–183, 1991
27. Hogan Q: Cardiovascular response to sympathetic block by regional anesthesia. Reg Anesth 21:26–34, 1997
28. Mulcahy D, Keegan J, Cunningham D, Quyyumi A, Crean P, Park A, Wright C, Fox K: Circadian variation of total ischaemic burden and its alteration with anti-anginal agents. Lancet 2:755–759, 1988
29. Willich SN, Pohjola Sintonen S, Bhatia SJ, Shook TL, Tofler GH,

Muller JE, Curtis DG, Williams GH, Stone PH: Suppression of silent ischemia by metoprolol without alteration of morning increase of platelet aggregability in patients with stable coronary artery disease. Circulation 79:557–565, 1989

30. Rocco MB, Barry J, Campbell S, Nabel E, Cook EF, Goldman L, Selwyn AP: Circadian variation of transient myocardial ischemia in patients with coronary artery disease. Circulation 75:395–400, 1987

31. Dorman BH, Zucker JR, Verrier ED, Gartman DM, Slachman FN: Clonidine improves perioperative myocardial ischemia, reduces anesthetic requirement, and alters hemodynamic parameters in patients undergoing coronary artery bypass surgery. J Cardiothorac Vasc Surg 7(4):386–395, 1993

32. β-blocker heart attack trial group: A randomized trial of propranolol in patients with acute myocardial infarction. II. Morbidity results. JAMA 250: 2814–2819, 1983

33. Klassen GA, Bramwell RS, Bromage PR, Zborowska Sluis DT: Effect of acute sympathectomy by epidural anesthesia on the canine coronary circulation. Anesthesiology 52:8–15, 1980

34. Groban L, Zvara DA, Deal DD, Vernon JC, Carpenter RL: Thoracic epidural anesthesia reduces infarct size in a canine model of myocardial ischemia and reperfusion injury. J Cardiothorac Vasc Anesth 13:579–585., 1999

35. Blomberg S, Curelaru I, Emanuelsson H, Herlitz J, Ponten J, Ricksten SE: Thoracic epidural anaesthesia in patients with unstable angina pectoris. Eur Heart J 10:437–444, 1989

36. Blomberg SG: Long-term home self-treatment with high thoracic epidural anesthesia in patients with severe coronary artery disease. Anesth-Analg 79:413–421, 1994

37. Tsuchida H, Omote T, Miyamoto M, Namiki A, Ichihara K, Abiko Y: Effects of thoracic epidural anesthesia on myocardial pH and metabolism during ischemia. Acta Anaesthesiol Scand 35:508–512, 1991

38. Hotvedt R, Platou ES, Refsum H: Electrophysiological effects of thoracic epidural anesthesia in the dog heart in situ. Cardiovasc Res 17:259–266, 1983

39. Sato K, Yamamura T, Murakami F, Yokota S, Kemmotsu O: Thoracic epidural anaesthesia combined with enflurane anaesthesia reduces atrioventricular conduction in dogs. Can J Anaesth 37:813–818, 1990

40. Kamibayashi T, Hayashi Y, Mammoto T, Yamatodani A, Taenaka N, Yoshiya I: Thoracic epidural anesthesia attenuates halothane-induced myocardial sensitization to dysrhythmogenic effect of epinephrine in dogs. Anesthesiology 82:129–134, 1995

41. Blomberg S, Ricksten SE: Thoracic epidural anaesthesia decreases

the incidence of ventricular arrhythmias during acute myocardial ischaemia in the anaesthetized rat. Acta Anaesthesiol Scand 32:173–178, 1988

42. Meissner A, Eckhardt L, Kirchhof P, Weber T, Rolf N, Breithardt G, Van Aken H, Haverkamp W: Effects of thoracic epidural anesthesia with and without autonomic nervous system blockade on cardiac monophasic action potentials and effective refractoriness in awake dogs. Anesthesiology 95:132–138, 2001

43. Rosenfeld BA, Beattie C, Christopherson R, Norris EJ, Frank SM, Breslow MJ, Rock P, Parker SD, Gottlieb SO, Perler BA, et al: The effects of different anesthetic regimens on fibrinolysis and the development of postoperative arterial thrombosis. Perioperative Ischemia Randomized Anesthesia Trial Study Group. Anesthesiology 79:435–443, 1993

44. Steele SM, Slaughter TF, Greenberg CS, Reves JG: Epidural anesthesia and analgesia: implications for perioperative coagulability. Anesth Analg 73:683–685, 1991

45. Christopherson R, Beattie C, Frank SM, Norris EJ, Meinert CL, Gottlieb SO, Yates H, Rock P, Parker SD, Perler BA, et al: Perioperative morbidity in patients randomized to epidural or general anesthesia for lower extremity vascular surgery. Perioperative Ischemia Randomized Anesthesia Trial Study Group. Anesthesiology 79:422–434, 1993

46. Tuman KJ, McCarthy RJ, March RJ, DeLaria GA, Patel RV, Ivankovich AD: Effects of epidural anesthesia and analgesia on coagulation and outcome after major vascular surgery. Anesth Analg 73:696–704, 1991

47. Henny CP, Odoom JA, ten Cate H, ten Cate JW, Oosterhoff RJ, Dabhoiwala NF, Sih IL: Effects of extradural bupivacaine on the haemostatic system. Br J Anaesth 58:301–305, 1986

48. Feinstein MG, Fiekers J, Fraser C: An analysis of the mechanism of local anesthetic inhibition of platelet aggregation and secretion. J Pharmacol Exp Ther 197:215–228, 1976

49. Nielsen T, Nielsen H, Husted S, Hansen S, Olsen K, Fjeldborg N: Stress response and platelet function in minor surgery during epidural bupivacaine and general anesthesia: effect of epidural morphine addition. Eur J Anaesthesiol 6:409–417, 1989

50. Modig J, Malmberg P, Karlstrom G: Effect of epidural versus general anaesthesia on calf blood flow. Acta Anaesthesiol Scand 24:305–309, 1980

51. Lundin S, Kirnö K, Wallin B, Elam M: Intraneural recording of muscle sympathetic activty during epidural anesthesia in humans. Anesth Analg 69:788–793, 1989

52. Hogan Q, Stadnicka A, Stekiel T, Bosnjak Z, Kampine J: Effects of

epidural and systemic lidocaine activity and mesenteric circulation in rabbits. Anesthesiology 79:1250–1260, 1993

53. Hogan Q, Stadnicka A, Stekiel T, Bosnjak Z, Kampine J: Region of epidural blockade determines sympathetic and mesenteric capacitance effects in rabbits. Anesthesiology 83:604–610, 1995

54. Mark AL: The Bezold-Jarisch reflex revisited: clinical implications of inhibitory reflexes originating in the heart. J Am Coll Cardiol 1:90–102, 1983

55. Mergner GW, Stolte AL, Frame WB, Lim HJ: Combined epidural analgesia and general anesthesia induce ischemia distal to a severe coronary artery stenosis in swine. Anesth Analg 78:37–45, 1994

56. Baron JF, Payen D, Coriat P, Edouard A, Viars P: Forearm vascular tone and reactivity during lumbar epidural anesthesia. Anesth Analg 67:1065–1070, 1988

57. Bonica JJ, Berges PU, Morikawa K: Circulatory effects of peridural block. I. Effects of level of analgesia and dose of lidocaine. Anesthesiology 33:619–626, 1970

58. Arndt JO, Hocck A, Stanton-Hicks M, Stuhmeier KO: Peridural anesthesia and the distribution of blood in supine humans. Anesthesiology 63:616–623, 1985

59. Taniguchi M, Kasaba T, Takasaki M: Epidural anesthesia enhances sympathetic nerve activity in the unanesthetized segments in cats. Anesth Analg 84:391–397, 1997

60. Saada M, Duval AM, Bonnet F, Rey B, Castillon G, Macquin Mavier I, Cabrit R, Boico O, Castaigne A: Abnormalities in myocardial segmental wall motion during lumbar epidural anesthesia. Anesthesiology 71:26–32, 1989

61. Rodgers A, Walker N, Schug S, McKee A, Kehlet H, van Zundert A, Sage D, Futter M, Saville G, Clark T, MacMahon S: Reduction of postoperative mortality and morbidity with epidural or spinal anaesthesia: Results from overview of randomised trials. Br Med J 321:1493, 2000

62. Yeager MP, Glass DD, Neff RK, Brinck Johnsen T: Epidural anesthesia and analgesia in high-risk surgical patients. Anesthesiology 66:729–736, 1987

63. Baron JF, Bertrand M, Barre E, Godet G, Mundler O, Coriat P, Viars P: Combined epidural and general anesthesia versus general anesthesia for abdominal aortic surgery. Anesthesiology 75:611–618, 1991

64. Bode RH, Jr., Lewis KP, Zarich SW, Pierce ET, Roberts M, Kowalchuk GJ, Satwicz PR, Gibbons GW, Hunter JA, Espanola CC, Nesto RW: Cardiac outcome after peripheral vascular surgery. Comparison of general and regional anesthesia. Anesthesiology 84:3–13, 1996

65. Sprung J, Lesitsky MA, Jagetia A, Tucker C, Saffian M, Gottlieb A: Cardiac arrest caused by coronary spasm in two patients during recovery from epidural anesthesia. Reg Anesth 21:253–260, 1996
66. Dureuil B, Viires N, Cantineau JP, Aubier M, Desmonts JM: Diaphragmatic contractility after upper abdominal surgery. J Appl Physiol 61:1775–1780, 1986
67. Ford GT, Whitelaw WA, Rosenal TW, Cruse PJ, Guenter CA: Diaphragm function after upper abdominal surgery in humans. Am Rev Respir Dis 127:431–436, 1983
68. Road JD, Burgess KR, Whitelaw WA, Ford GT: Diaphragm function and respiratory response after upper abdominal surgery in dogs. J Appl Physiol 57:576–582, 1984
69. Easton PA, Fitting JW, Arnoux R, Guerraty A, Grassino AE: Recovery of diaphragm function after laparotomy and chronic sonomicrometer implantation. J Appl Physiol 66: 613–621, 1989
70. Rosenberg J, Rasmussen V, Jessen Fv, Ullstad T, Kehlet H: Late postoperative episodic and constant hypoxaemia and associated ECG abnormalities. Br J Anaesth 65: 684–691, 1990
71. Beydon L, Hassapopoulos J, Quera MA, Rauss A, Becquemin JP, Bonnet F, Harf A, Goldenberg F: Risk factors for oxygen desaturation during sleep, after abdominal surgery. Br J Anaesth 69:137–142, 1992
72. Catley DM, Thornton C, Jordan C, Tech B, Lehane JR, Royston D, Jones JG: Pronounced, episodic oxygen desaturation in the postoperative period: its association with ventilatory pattern and analgesic regimen. Anesthesiology 63:20–28, 1985
73. Slinger P, Shennib H, Wilson S: Postthoracotomy pulmonary function: a comparison of epidural versus intravenous meperidine infusions. J Cardiothorac Vasc Anesth 9:128–134, 1995
74. Guinard JP, Mavrocordato P, Chiolero P, Carpenter RL: A randomized comparison of intravenous versus lumbar and thoracic epidural fentanyl for analgesia after thoracotomy. Anesthesiology 77:1108–1115, 1992
75. Simonneau G, Vivien A, Sartene R, Kunstlinger F, Samii K, Noviant Y, Duroux P: Diaphragm dysfunction induced by upper abdominal surgery. Role of postoperative pain. Am Rev Respir Dis 128:899–903, 1983
76. Bonnet F, Blery C, Zatan M, Simonet O, Brage D, Gaudy J: Effect of epidural morphine on post-operative pulmonary dysfunction. Acta Anaesthesiol Scand 28:147–151, 1984
77. Spence AA, Smith G: Postoperative analgesia and lung function: a comparison of morphine with extradural block. Br J Anaesth 43:144–148, 1971
78. Polaner DM, Kimball WR, Fratacci MD, Wain JC, Zapol WM: Tho-

racic epidural anesthesia increases diaphragmatic shortening after thoracotomy in the awake lamb. Anesthesiology 79:808–816, 1993

79. Mankikian B, Cantineau JP, Bertrand M, Kieffer E, Sartene R, Viars P: Improvement of diaphragmatic function by a thoracic extradural block after upper abdominal surgery. Anesthesiology 68:379–386, 1988

80. Fratacci MD, Kimball WR, Wain JC, Kacmarek RM, Polaner DM, Zapol WM: Diaphragmatic shortening after thoracic surgery in humans. Effects of mechanical ventilation and thoracic epidural anesthesia. Anesthesiology 79:654–665, 1993

81. Lundh R, Hedenstierna G, Johansson H: Ventilation-perfusion relationships during epidural analgesia. Acta Anaesthesiol Scand 27:410–416, 1983

82. Sakura S, Saito Y, Kosaka Y: The effects of epidural anesthesia on ventilatory response to hypercapnia and hypoxia in elderly patients. Anesth Analg 82:306–311, 1996

83. Warner D, Warner M, Ritman E: Human chest wall function during epidural anesthesia. Anesthesiology 85:761–773, 1996

84. Theissen IL, Meißner A: Hypoxic pulmonary vasoconstriction. Anaesthesist 45:643–652, 1996

85. Ishibe Y, Shiokawa Y, Umeda T, Uno H, Nakamura M, Izumi T: The effect of thoracic epidural anesthesia on hypoxic pulmonary vasoconstriction in dogs: an analysis of the pressure-flow curve. Anesth Analg 82: 1049–1055, 1996

86. Liu S, Carpenter RL, Neal JM: Epidural anesthesia and analgesia. Their role in postoperative outcome. Anesthesiology 82:1474–1506, 1995

87. Gelman S: General versus regional anesthesia for peripheral vascular surgery—is the problem solved? Anesthesiology 79:415–418, 1993

88. Go AS, Browner WS: Cardiac outcomes after regional anesthesia—Do we have the answer? Anesthesiology 84:1–2, 1996

Mark A. Chaney, M.D.

Intrathecal Techniques for Adult Cardiac
3 | Surgery

INTRODUCTION

Inadequate analgesia and/or an uninhibited stress response during the postoperative period may lead to many adverse hemodynamic, metabolic, immunologic, and hemostatic alterations (1–3). Aggressive control of postoperative pain with regional anesthesia and analgesia, associated with an attenuated stress response, may decrease morbidity and mortality in high-risk patients after noncardiac surgery (4, 5). Aggressive control of postoperative pain with intravenous (IV) analgesics, associated with an attenuated stress response in patients after cardiac surgery, may also decrease morbidity and mortality (6, 7). The perioperative use of intrathecal (IT) or epidural (EPI) anesthesia and analgesia in patients undergoing cardiac surgery may beneficially affect outcome by producing intense postoperative analgesia, stress-response attenuation, and thoracic cardiac sympathectomy (8). However, the technique can be associated with undesirable drug effects that may possibly increase morbidity, and it entails an increased risk of hematoma formation (8). This chapter summarizes the risks and benefits associated with the application of IT anesthesia and analgesia in patients undergoing cardiac surgery and suggests future directions for investigation.

POTENTIAL BENEFITS

In patients undergoing cardiac surgery, perioperative myocardial ischemia (diagnosed by electrocardiography and/or transesophageal

Regional Anesthesia for Cardiothoracic Surgery, edited by Mark Chaney,
Lippincott Williams & Wilkins, Baltimore © 2002.

echocardiography) is most commonly observed during the immediate postoperative period (25%–38% incidence) and is related to outcome (9, 10). Intraoperatively, initiation of cardiopulmonary bypass (CPB) causes significant increases in stress-response hormones (nonepinephrine, epinephrine, etc.) that persist into the immediate postoperative period and may contribute to myocardial ischemia observed during this time (11–13). Furthermore, postoperative myocardial ischemia may be aggravated by cardiac sympathetic nerve activation, which disrupts the balance between coronary blood flow and myocardial oxygen demand (14). During the pivotal immediate postoperative period after cardiac surgery, the major potential benefits offered by IT anesthesia and analgesia are intense analgesia, stress-response attenuation, and thoracic cardiac sympathectomy.

Intense Postoperative Analgesia

Aggressive control of postoperative pain in patients after cardiac surgery may beneficially affect outcome. In adults undergoing coronary artery bypass grafting (CABG), intense analgesia (continuous IV sufentanil infusion) during the immediate postoperative period (first 18 hours) decreases the incidence and severity of myocardial ischemia as diagnosed by the electrocardiography (6). In neonates undergoing cardiac surgery, intense analgesia (continuous IV fentanyl or sufentanil infusion) during the immediate postoperative period (first 24 hours) decreases morbidity and mortality (7). Unfortunately, aggressive control of pain with IV opioids in this manner does not allow tracheal extubation to occur in the immediate postoperative period. IT anesthesia and analgesia is an attractive alternative to IV opioids in this setting for its potential to produce intense analgesia yet still allow extubation to occur in the immediate postoperative period.

Stress Response Attenuation

An uninhibited stress response during the postoperative period may lead to many adverse hemodynamic (tachycardia, hypertension, vasoconstriction), metabolic (increased catabolism), immunologic (impaired immune response), and hemostatic (platelet activation) alterations (1–3). IT anesthesia and analgesia (with local anesthetics or opioids) can effectively inhibit the stress response associated with surgical procedures (14). Local anesthetics appear to possess greater efficacy than opioids in stress-response attenuation, perhaps because of their unique mechanism of action (14). Although still a matter of some debate, stress-response attenuation with EPI local anesthetics and/or opioids in high-risk patients after major noncardiac surgery may decrease morbidity and mortality (4, 5, 14). In patients undergoing cardiac surgery, initiation of CPB causes significant increases in stress-response hormones that persist into the immediate postoperative period (11–13). Attenuation of this component of the stress response with IV opioids may also decrease morbidity and mortality (6, 7). Unfortunately, stress-response attenuation in patients undergoing cardiac surgery with IV opioids in this manner does not allow extubation to occur in the immediate postoperative period. IT anesthesia and analgesia (particularly with local anesthetics) is an attractive alternative to IV opioids in this setting for its potential to attenuate the stress response yet still allow extubation to occur in the immediate postoperative period.

Thoracic Cardiac Sympathectomy

The myocardium and coronary vasculature are densely innervated by sympathetic nerve fibers that arise from T1 to T5 and profoundly influence total coronary blood flow and distribution (15). Cardiac sympathetic nerve activation initiates coronary artery vasoconstriction (16) and paradoxical vasoconstriction in response to intrinsic vasodilators (17). In patients with coronary artery disease, cardiac sympathetic nerve activation disrupts the normal matching of coronary blood flow and myocardial oxygen demand (18, 19). Animal models show an intense poststenotic vasoconstrictive mechanism mediated by cardiac sympathetic nerve activation that attenuates local metabolic vasodilation in response to myocardial ischemia (20, 21). Furthermore, myocardial ischemia initiates a cardiocardiac reflex mediated by sympathetic nerve fibers, which augments the ischemic process (22). Cardiac sympathetic nerve activation likely plays a central role in initiating postoperative myocardial ischemia by decreasing the myocardial oxygen supply via the mechanisms listed above (14, 23).

Thoracic EPI anesthesia with local anesthetics effectively blocks cardiac sympathetic nerve afferent and efferent fibers (14) and IT local anesthetics should have similar beneficial physiologic effects. Opioids, which are administered similarly, are unable to effectively block cardiac sympathetic nerve activity (14). Patients with symptomatic coronary artery disease benefit from cardiac sympathectomy, and the application of thoracic sympathetic blockade in the management of angina pectoris was described as early as 1965 (24). Thoracic EPI anesthesia with local anesthetics increases the diameter of stenotic epicardial coronary artery segments without causing dilation of coronary arterioles (18), decreases determinants of myocardial oxygen demand (19), improves left ventricular function (25), and decreases anginal symptoms (26, 27). Furthermore, cardiac sympathectomy increases the endocardial to epicardial blood flow ratio (28, 29), beneficially affects collateral blood flow during myocardial ischemia (29), decreases poststenotic vasconstriction (21), and attenuates the myocardial ischemia-induced cardiocardiac reflex (21). In an animal model, thoracic EPI anesthesia with local anesthetics decreases myocardial infarct size after coronary artery occlusion (28). Of note, these beneficial effects are not caused by systemic absorption of the local anesthetic (28). In short, thoracic EPI anesthesia with local anesthetics may benefit patients undergoing cardiac surgery by effectively blocking cardiac sympathetic nerve activity and improving the myocardial oxygen supply–demand balance.

CLINICAL UTILIZATION OF INTRATHECAL TECHNIQUES

Table 3–1 summarizes the clinical investigations detailing application of IT anesthesia and analgesia to patients undergoing cardiac surgery (30–54). Application of IT analgesia to patients undergoing cardiac surgery was initially reported by Mathews and Abrams in 1980 (54). They described the administration of IT morphine (1.5–4.0 mg) to 40 adults after the induction of anesthesia for cardiac surgery (54). Postoperatively, all 40 patients were entirely pain free for the first 27.5 hours, and 17 did not require any analgesics prior to discharge from the hospital (54). Of the 17 patients who received 4.0 mg of IT morphine, 11 required no postoperative analgesic drugs (54).

After this impressive display, others have subsequently applied IT anesthesia and analgesia to patients undergoing cardiac surgery (Table 3–1). Most have used IT morphine in hopes of providing prolonged postoperative analgesia. Some have used IT fentanyl, sufentanil, or local anesthetics for intraoperative anesthesia and analgesia (with stress-response attenuation) and/or thoracic cardiac sympathectomy.

Three randomized, blind, placebo-controlled studies demonstrate the ability of IT morphine to induce significant postoperative analgesia after cardiac surgery (30, 41, 48). In one study, patients were randomized to receive either IT morphine (4.0 mg) or IT placebo prior to the induction of anesthesia (41). Intraoperative anesthetic management was standardized, and after tracheal extubation, all received exclusively IV morphine via patient-controlled analgesia (41). Patients who received IT morphine required significantly less IV morphine than placebo controls (33.2 vs 51.1 mg, respectively) during the initial 48 postoperative hours (41). In another study, patients were randomized to receive either IT morphine (0.5 mg) or IT placebo prior to the induction of anesthesia

(48). Intraoperative anesthetic management was standardized and, postoperatively, all patients received exclusively IV morphine administered by a nurse who tried to keep the linear analog pain score at less than 4 (a score of 1 represented no pain, 10 represented the worst pain imaginable; the scale was 25 cm long) (48). Patients who received IT morphine required significantly less IV morphine than placebo controls (2.4 vs 8.3 mg, respectively) during the initial 30 hours after IT injection (48). In yet another study, patients were randomized to receive either IT morphine (250 µg or 500 µg) or IT placebo prior to induction of anesthesia (30). Intraoperative anesthetic management was standardized and, postoperatively, all patients received IV morphine as needed for pain (30). Patients who received IT morphine, 250 µg or 500 µg, required significantly less IV morphine than placebo controls (13.6 vs 11.7 vs 21.3 mg, respectively) during the initial 24 postoperative hours (30).

However, one randomized, blind, placebo-controlled study indicates that IT morphine may not induce reliable postoperative analgesia after cardiac surgery (38). In this study, patients were randomized to receive either IT morphine (10 µg/kg) or IT placebo prior to induction of anesthesia (38). Intraoperative anesthetic management was standardized and after tracheal extubation all received exclusively IV morphine via patient-controlled analgesia (38). Patients who received IT morphine actually required more IV morphine than placebo controls (49.8 vs 36.2 mg, respectively) during the first 48 hours after extubation although the difference was not statistically significant (38).

Numerous suboptimal studies (retrospective, observational, etc.) attest to the ability of IT morphine to induce substantial postoperative analgesia in patients after cardiac surgery (Table 3–1). Doses of 0.5 to 10.0 mg administered prior to CPB appears to initiate reliable postoperative analgesia, the quality of which depends not only on the dose administered but also on the type and amount of IV analgesics used for the intraoperative baseline anesthetic. The optimal dose of IT morphine for achieving the maximum postoperative analgesia with minimum undesirable drug effects is uncertain. Naturally, when larger doses of IT morphine are used, more intense and prolonged postoperative analgesia is purchased at the expense of more undesirable drug effects (47, 53).

Because of morphine's low lipid solubility, analgesic effects after IT injection are delayed. Thus, even large doses of IT morphine administered to patients before cardiac surgery do not initiate reliable intraoperative analgesia (48–50, 53) and therefore would not be expected to attenuate the stress response associated with CPB. Only an extremely large dose of IT morphine (10.0 mg) may initiate reliable intraoperative analgesia in this setting (52). Only one study has examined the ability of IT morphine to attenuate the stress response associated with CPB as measured by blood catecholamine levels (41). Patients were random-

TABLE 3.1.   Reports of Intrathecal Anesthesia and Analgesia for Cardiac Surgery

Author (reference)	Year	Study Design	Total Patients	Drugs: Dose	Intraoperative Management	Remarks
Alhashemi et al. (30)	2000	Prospective, randomized, blind, placebo-controlled	50	Morphine: 250 mcg or 500 mcg	Standardized	Significant postoperative analgesia
Latham et al. (31)	2000	Prospective, randomized	40	Morphine: 8 mcg/kg	Standardized	No benefit
Zarate et al. (32)	2000	Prospective randomized	40	Morphine: 8 mcg/kg	Standardized	Reliable postoperative analgesia
Bowler et al. (33)*	2000	Prospective, randomized	25	Morphine: 2.0 mg	Standardized	Reliable postoperative analgesia, facilitated early extubation
Lee et al. (34)*	2000	Prospective, randomized, blind, placebo-controlled	15	Bupivacaine: 37.5 mg	Standardized	No benefit
Peterson et al. (35)	2000	Retrospective	18	Morphine: 5–10 mcg/kg Tetracaine: 1–2 mg/kg	Not Standardized	No benefit
Hammer et al. (36)	2000	Retrospective	25	Morphine: 7–10 mcg/kg Tetracaine: 0.5–2 mg/kg	Not Standardized	No benefit
Djaiani et al. (37)*	2000	Prospective, randomized	24	Morphine: 2.0 mg	Standardized	Possible postoperative pulmonary benefits
Chaney et al. (38)	1999	Prospective, randomized, blind, placebo-controlled	40	Morphine: 10 mcg/kg	Standardized	No benefit
Shroff et al. (39)	1997	Prospective, randomized	21	Morphine: 10 mcg/kg Fentanyl: 25 mcg	Not Standardized	Reliable postoperative analgesia, facilitated early extubation
Chaney et al. (40)	1997	Prospective, randomized, blind, placebo-controlled	40	Morphine: 10 mcg/kg	Standardized	Hindered early extubation
Chaney et al. (41)	1996	Prospective, randomized, blind, placebo-controlled	60	Morphine: 4.0 mg	Standardized	Significant postoperative analgesia, no stress-response attenuation
Kowalewski et al. (42)	1996	Case report	1	Morphine: 0.5 mg Bupivacaine: 30 mg	NA	Facilitated early extubation
Taylor et al. (43)	1996	Retrospective	152	Morphine: 30 mcg/kg	Not Standardized	Reliable postoperative analgesia

Author (reference)	Year	Study design	N	Drug: dose	Standardization	Outcome
Kowalewski et al. (44)	1994	Retrospective	18	Morphine: 0.5–1.0 mg; Bupivacaine: 23–30 mg; Lidocaine: 150 mg	Not Standardized	Reliable postoperative analgesia, possible thoracic cardiac sympathectomy
Swenson et al. (45)	1994	Retrospective	10	Morphine: 0.5 mg; Sufentanil: 50 mcg	Not Standardized	Reliable postoperative analgesia, facilitated early extubation
Shroff and Bishop (46)*	1994	Prospective, randomized	20	Morphine: 10 mcg/kg; Fentanyl: 25 mcg	Not Standardized	Reliable postoperative analgesia
Fitzpatrick and Moriarty (47)	1988	Prospective, randomized	44	Morphine: 1.0–2.0 mg	Not Standardized	Significant postoperative analgesia
Vanstrum et al. (48)	1988	Prospective, randomized, blind, placebo-controlled	30	Morphine: 0.5 mg	Standardized	Significant postoperative analgesia, possible stress-response attenuation
Casey et al. (49)	1987	Prospective, randomized, blind, placebo-controlled	40	Morphine: 20 mcg/kg	Standardized	No benefit
Cheun (50)	1987	Prospective, observational	180	Morphine: 0.1 mg/kg; Meperidine: 1.5 mg/kg	Not Standardized	Reliable postoperative analgesia
Aun et al. (51)	1985	Prospective, randomized	60	Morphine: 2.0–4.0 mg	Not Standardized	Significant postoperative analgesia
Vincenty et al. (52)*	1985	Prospective, observational	20	Morphine: 10.0 mg	Not Standardized	Reliable postoperative analgesia, possible stress-response attenuation
Jones et al. (53)	1984	Prospective, observational	56	Morphine: 20–30 mcg/kg	Not Standardized	Reliable postoperative analgesia
Mathews and Abrams (54)+	1980	Retrospective	40	Morphine: 1.5–4.0 mg	Not Standardized	Reliable postoperative analgesia

* = Abstract
+ = Correspondence
mcg = micrograms
mg = milligrams
kg = kilograms
NA = not applicable

ized to receive either IT morphine (4.0 mg) or IT placebo prior to the induction of anesthesia (41). Intraoperative anesthetic management was standardized, and arterial blood samples were obtained perioperatively to ascertain norepinephrine and epinephrine levels (41). Patients who were administered IT morphine experienced similar perioperative increases in blood catecholamine levels when compared with placebo controls (41).

Although unable to attenuate the stress response associated with CPB, IT morphine (by initiating postoperative analgesia) may attenuate the stress response during the immediate postoperative period (48). Patients who were administered 0.5 mg of IT morphine prior to the induction of anesthesia not only required significantly less IV morphine postoperatively than placebo controls but also required significantly less IV nitroprusside (58.1 vs 89.1 mg, respectively) during the initial 24 postoperative hours to control hypertension, which suggests partial stress-response attenuation (48).

Some investigators have used IT fentanyl, sufentanil, or local anesthetics, hoping to provide intraoperative anesthesia and analgesia (and stress-response attenuation), with mixed results (Table 3–1). Administration of IT local anesthetics to patients after the induction of anesthesia for cardiac surgery may help promote intraoperative hemodynamic stability (42, 44), whereas IT sufentanil (50 µg) administered prior to the induction of anesthesia for cardiac surgery can reduce volatile anesthetic requirements during mediastinal dissection but is unable to reliably block hemodyamic responses to laryngoscopy and intubation (45).

Most attempts at inducing thoracic cardiac sympathectomy in patients undergoing cardiac surgery have utilized thoracic EPI anesthesia with local anesthetics (8). Only two groups of investigators have attempted cardiac sympathectomy in this setting with an IT injection of local anesthetics. As reviewed retrospectively in 1994 by Kowalewski et al, 18 adult patients were administered lumbar IT hyperbaric bupivacaine (23–30 mg) and/or hyperbaric lidocaine (150 mg) mixed with morphine (0.5–1.0 mg) after the induction of anesthesia (44). In an attempt to produce a total spinal and, thus, thoracic cardiac sympathectomy, Trendelenburg position was maintained for at least 10 minutes after the IT injection (44). Heart rate decreased significantly (baseline mean 67 beats per minute to postinjection mean 52 beats per minute) after injection (indicating cardiac sympathectomy was obtained), and no patient exhibited electrocardiographic evidence of myocardial ischemia prior to CPB (44). Although the authors report that the technique provided stable perioperative hemodynamics, 17 of 18 patients required IV phenylephrine at some time intraoperatively to increase blood pressure (44). The same group reported in 1996 similar hemodynamic changes that occurred in a 10-year-old child with Kawasaki's disease who underwent CABG after receiving IT hyperbaric bupivacaine mixed with morphine via a lumbar puncture after induction of anesthesia (42). More recently, Lee et al, in abstract form, described their experience with induction of high spinal anesthesia in patients undergoing cardiac surgery (34). They administered 37.5 mg of hyperbaric bupivacaine to 8 patients prior to induction of anesthesia for cardiac surgery (7 patients received sham spinal) (34). Like the Kowalewski group, they maintained Trendelenburg position following the IT injection, and IV phenylephrine was used to maintain blood pressure (34). They report that the technique of high spinal anesthesia for cardiac surgery is "safe and effective," yet patients receiving IT bupivacaine required significantly more phenylephrine then the sham spinal patients to maintain blood pressure prior to CPB (610 ± 525 mcg vs 136 ± 217 mcg, respectively, $p = 0.03$) (34). There were no differences between the two groups regarding postoperative cortisol and cardiac enzyme levels, postoperative morphine utilization, postoperative pulmonary function, or extubation time (34).

In summary, the administration of IT morphine to patients prior to CPB appears to initiate reliable postoperative analgesia after cardiac surgery. IT opioids or local anesthetics cannot reliably attenuate the stress response associated with CPB that persists during the immediate postoperative period. Although IT local anesthetics (not opioids) may induce thoracic cardiac sympathectomy, the hemodynamic changes associated with a total spinal make the technique unpalatable.

Clinical Outcome

All reports of IT anesthesia and analgesia for cardiac surgery involve small numbers of patients and few are well-designed (Table 3–1). Only seven studies involving IT anesthesia and analgesia are prospective randomized, blind, and placebo-controlled (one being published only in abstract form). Furthermore, none of these investigations uses clinical outcome as a primary end point. Thus, there are clear deficiencies in the literature that prohibit definitive analysis of the risk–benefit ratio of IT anesthesia and analgesia for cardiac surgery.

UNDESIRABLE DRUG EFFECTS

Opioids

Although many have been described, the four clinically relevant undesirable drug effects of IT opioids are pruritus, nausea and vomiting, urinary retention, and respiratory depression (55). After administration of

IT opioids, the most common side effect is pruritus. The incidence varies widely, from 0% to 100%, and is often identified only after direct questioning of patients. Severe pruritus is rare, occurring in only approximately 1% of patients. The incidence of nausea and vomiting is approximately 30%. The incidence of urinary retention varies widely, from 0% to 80%, and occurs most frequently in young male patients.

When IT opioids are used in patients undergoing cardiac surgery, the incidence of pruritus, nausea and vomiting, and urinary retention is similar to that described above (40, 41, 43, 47–51,53). Of note, if a large dose (4.0 mg) of IT morphine is administered, prolonged postoperative urinary retention may occur (41).

The most important undesirable drug effect of IT opioids is respiratory depression. Only 4 months after the initial use of IT (56) and EPI (57) opioids in humans in 1979, life-threatening respiratory depression was reported (58–60). The incidence of respiratory depression that requires intervention after conventional doses of IT opioids is approximately 1%, the same as that after conventional doses of intramuscular and IV opioids. Early respiratory depression occurs within minutes of opioid injection and is associated with administration of IT fentanyl or sufentanil. Delayed respiratory depression occurs hours after opioid injection and is associated with administration of IT morphine. Delayed respiratory depression results from cephalad migration of morphine in cerebrospinal fluid and the subsequent stimulation of opioid receptors located in the ventral medulla (61). Factors that increase the risk of respiratory depression include large and/or repeated doses of opioids, intrathecal utilization, advanced age, and concomitant use of IV sedatives (55).

The magnitude of postoperative respiratory depression is profoundly influenced by the dose of IT morphine administered and the type and amount of IV analgesics and amnestics used for the intraoperative baseline anesthetic. Prolonged postoperative respiratory depression may delay tracheal extubation (38, 40, 41), and naloxone may be required in some patients (43, 47, 53). Children may be more susceptible to developing postoperative respiratory depression when IT morphine is used in this setting (53). Of 56 children (aged 1–17 years) administered either 20 or 30 μg/kg IT morphine prior to surgical incision, 3 of 29 who received 20 μg/kg and 6 of 27 receiving 30 μg/kg required naloxone postoperatively for respiratory depression (53).

One prospective, randomized, blind, placebo-controlled study indicates that administration of IT morphine to patients undergoing cardiac surgery may be contraindicated if early extubation is planned (40). Patients were randomized to receive either IT morphine (10 μg/kg) or IT placebo prior to the induction of anesthesia (40). Intraoperative anesthetic management was standardized and consisted of IV fentanyl (20 μg/kg) and midazolam (10 mg, total), along with inhaled isoflurane and/or IV nitroglycerin, if required (40). Regarding patients extubated during the immediate postoperative period, the mean time from intensive care unit arrival to extubation was significantly increased in those who received IT morphine compared with those who received IT placebo (10.9 vs 7.6 hours, respectively) (40). An extension of this study by the same group of investigators revealed that decreasing the amounts of intravenous agents administered intraoperatively allowed for equivalent extubation times (38). In this second study, patients were randomized to receive either IT morphine (10 µg/kg) or IT placebo prior to induction of anesthesia (38). Intraoperative anesthetic management was standardized and consisted of IV fentanyl (10 µg/kg) and midazolam (0.20 mg/kg), along with inhaled isoflurane and/or IV nitroglycerin, if required (38). Of the patients tracheally extubated during the immediate postoperative period (within 12 hours), mean time to extubation was similar in patients who received IT morphine (6.8 hours) or IT placebo (6.5 hours) (38). However, four patients who received IT morphine had extubation substantially delayed (>12 hours) because of prolonged ventilatory depression (38). Another prospective, randomized, blind, placebo-controlled study indicates that IT morphine may not reliably facilitate early extubation following cardiac surgery (30). In this study, patients were randomized to receive either IT morphine (250 µg or 500 µg) or IT placebo prior to the induction of anesthesia (30). Intraoperative anesthetic management was standardized and consisted of IV fentanyl (15 µg/kg) and midazolam (20 µg/kg), along with inhaled isoflurane and/or IV propofol, if required (30). The mean time from intensive care unit arrival to extubation in patients receiving IT morphine, 250 µg or 500 µg, was equivalent to placebo controls (325 vs 409 vs 441 minutes, respectively) (30). However, other less well-designed studies indicate that IT morphine may yet prove to be a useful adjunct for cardiac surgery and early extubation (42, 45). The optimal dose of IT morphine in this setting, along with the optimal intraoperative baseline anesthetic, that will provide significant analgesia yet not delay tracheal extubation in the immediate postoperative period remains to be elucidated.

Local Anesthetics

The most troubling and undesirable drug effect of IT local anesthetics is hypotension. Spinal anesthesia to upper thoracic dermatomes produces a decrease in mean arterial blood pressure that is accompanied by a parallel decrease in coronary blood flow (62, 63). Exactly what percentage of blood pressure decrease is acceptable remains speculative, especially in patients with coronary artery disease. Disturbances in myocardial oxygenation occur in patients with coronary artery disease if coronary perfusion pressure is allowed to decrease by more than 50% during induction of thoracic EPI anesthesia with local anesthetics (64). Furthermore, if alpha adrenergic agonists are used to increase blood pressure, there may be detrimental effects (vasoconstriction) on the native coronary arteries and bypass grafts (65, 66). Of the 27 patients who received IT local anesthetics to produce a total spinal for cardiac surgery, 26 required IV phenylephrine intraoperatively to increase blood pressure, which indicates that hypotension is a substantial problem with this technique (34, 42, 44).

RISK OF HEMATOMA FORMATION

IT instrumentation entails risk, the most feared complication being epidural hematoma formation. The estimated incidence of hematoma formation is approximately 1:220,000 after IT injection (67). Hematoma formation is more common (approximately 1:150,000) after EPI instrumentation because larger needles are used, catheters are placed, and the venous plexus in the EPI space is prominent (67). Furthermore, hematoma formation does not occur exclusively during EPI catheter insertion; almost half of all cases develop after catheter removal (67).

Although spontaneous hematomas can occur in the absence of IT instrumentation (68), most occur when IT instrumentation is performed in a patient with a coagulopathy (from any cause) or when instrumentation is difficult or traumatic (67). Paradoxically, IT or EPI instrumentation has been performed safely in patients with known coagulopathy (69, 70). Of 1000 epidural catheterizations performed in 950 patients receiving oral anticoagulants at time of catheter insertion, none developed signs or symptoms of hematoma formation (70). Of 336 epidural injections performed in 36 patients with chronic cancer pain either fully anticoagulated (oral anticoagulants or IV heparin) or profoundly thrombocytopenic (platelet count $<50,000/mm^3$) at the time of instrumentation, none developed signs or symptoms of hematoma formation (69).

Risk is increased when IT instrumentation is performed prior to systemic heparinization, and hematoma formation has occurred in patients when diagnostic or therapeutic lumbar puncture has been followed by systemic heparinization (71–74). When lumbar puncture is followed by systemic heparinization, concurrent use of aspirin, difficult or traumatic instrumentation, and administration of IV heparin within 1 hour of instrumentation increases the risk of hematoma formation (73). However, by observing certain precautions, IT instrumentation can be performed safely in patients who will subsequently receive IV heparin (75, 76). By delaying surgery 24 hours in the event of a traumatic tap, by delaying heparinization 60 minutes after catheter insertion, and by maintaining tight perioperative control of anticoagulation, more than 4000 IT or EPI catheterizations were performed safely in patients undergoing peripheral vascular surgery who received IV heparin after catheter insertion (76). A retrospective review involving 912 patients further indicates that EPI catheterization prior to systematic heparinization for peripheral vascular surgery is safe (75). However, the magnitude of anticoagulation in these two studies, activated partial thromboplastin time approximately 100 seconds (75) and activated clotting time approximately twice the baseline value (76), involving patients undergoing peripheral vascular surgery was significantly less than the degree of anticoagulation required in patients subjected to CPB.

Most studies investigating the use of IT anesthesia and analgesia in patients undergoing cardiac surgery include precautions to decrease risk of hematoma formation. Some used the technique only after the demonstration of laboratory evidence of normal coagulation parameters, delayed surgery 24 hours in the event of traumatic tap, or required that the time from instrumentation to systemic heparinization exceed 60 minutes. In studies utilizing EPI catheters, most inserted catheters the day before scheduled surgery.

Although hematoma formation has never been reported in a patient receiving IT instrumentation prior to systemic heparinization required for CPB, the risk may be as high as 0.35% (71). A recently published extensive mathematical analysis by Ho et al of the approximately 10,840 IT injections in patients subjected to systemic heparinization required for CPB (without a single episode of hematoma formation) reported in the literature as of the year 2000 estimated that the minimum risk of hematoma formation was 1:220,000 and the maximum risk of hematoma formation was 1:3,600 (95% confidence level), yet the maximum risk may be as high as 1:2,400 (99% confidence level) (77). Certain precautions, however, may decrease the risk (67, 71). The technique should not be used in a patient with known coagulopathy from any cause. Surgery should be delayed 24 hours in the event of a traumatic tap, and time from instrumentation to systemic heparinization should exceed 60 minutes. Additionally, heparin effect and reversal should be tightly controlled (smallest amount of heparin for the shortest duration compatible with therapeutic objectives), and patients should be closely monitored postoperatively for signs and symptoms of hematoma formation. An obvious economic disadvantage of IT instrumentation in patients prior to cardiac surgery is the possible delay in surgery in the event of a traumatic tap.

SUMMARY AND FUTURE DIRECTIONS

The potential benefits offered by IT anesthesia and analgesia for cardiac surgery include intense postoperative analgesia, stress-response attenuation, and thoracic cardiac sympathectomy. IT anesthesia and analgesia with opioids or local anesthetics may induce reliable postoperative analgesia in patients after cardiac surgery. Significant stress-response attenuation and thoracic cardiac sympathectomy are reliably achieved in this setting only with EPI administration of local anesthetics. The most important undesirable drug effect of opioids used in this manner is respiratory depression, which may delay postoperative tracheal extubation, whereas for local anesthetics, it is hypotension, which may decrease coronary blood flow. Although never reported in a patient receiving IT or EPI instrumentation prior to systemic heparinization required for CPB, the risk of hematoma formation is increased, and certain precautions should be observed.

It is not clear whether intense postoperative analgesia, stress-response attenuation, and/or thoracic cardiac sympathectomy in patients undergoing cardiac surgery affect outcome. All reports of IT anesthesia and analgesia for cardiac surgery involve small numbers of patients; few are well-designed, and none uses clinical outcome as a primary end point. Thus, there are clear deficiencies in the literature that prohibit definitive analysis of the risk–benefit ratio of IT anesthesia and analgesia for cardiac surgery. Despite this, a recently published anonymous survey of members of the Society of Cardiovascular Anesthesiologists by Goldstein et al indicates that almost 8% of practicing anesthesiologists incorporate IT techniques into their anesthetic management of adults undergoing cardiac surgery (78). Of these anesthesiologists, 75% practice in the United States, 72% perform the IT injection prior to induction of anesthesia, 97% utilize morphine, 13% utilize fentanyl, 2% utilize sufentanil, 10% utilize lidocaine, and 3% utilize tetracaine (78). Future directions in this fertile area should focus on development of well-designed studies with adequate numbers of patients that investigate the ability of IT anesthesia and analgesia to affect morbidity and mortality in patients after cardiac surgery. Furthermore, the optimal dose of IT morphine used in this setting, along with the optimal intraoperative baseline anesthetic that will provide significant analgesia yet not delay tracheal extubation in the immediate postoperative period, remains to be elucidated. Only after such studies are performed will a definitive analysis of the risk–benefit ratio of IT anesthesia and analgesia for cardiac surgery be possible.

References

1. Weissman C: The metabolic response to stress: An overview and update (review article). Anesthesiology 73:308–327, 1990
2. Kehlet H: Surgical stress: The role of pain and analgesia (review article). Br J Anaesth 63:189–195, 1989

3. Roizen MF: Should we all have a sympathectomy at birth? Or at least preoperatively? (editorial). Anesthesiology 68:482–484, 1988
4. Tuman KJ, McCarthy RJ, March RJ, et al: Effects of epidural anesthesia and analgesia on coagulation and outcome after major vascular surgery. Anesth Analg 73:696–704,1991
5. Yeager MP, Glass DD, Neff RK, Brinck-Johnson T: Epidural anesthesia and analgesia in high-risk surgical patients. Anesthesiology 66:729–736, 1987
6. Mangano DT, Siliciano D, Hollenberg M, et al: Postoperative myocardial ischemia: Therapeutic trials using intensive analgesia following surgery. Anesthesiology 76:342–353, 1992
7. Anand KJS, Hickey PR: Halothane-morphine compared with high-dose sufentanil for anesthesia and postoperative analgesia in neonatal cardiac surgery. N Engl J Med 326:1–9, 1992
8. Chaney MA: Intrathecal and epidural anesthesia and analgesia for cardiac surgery (review article). Anesth Analg 84:1211–1221, 1997
9. Smith RC, Leung JM, Mangano DT, SPI Research Group: Postoperative myocardial ischemia in patients undergoing coronary artery bypass graft surgery. Anesthesiology 74:464–473, 1991
10. Leung JM, O'Kelly B, Browner WS, et al: Prognostic importance of postbypass regional wall-motion abnormalities in patients undergoing coronary artery bypass graft surgery. Anesthesiology 71:16–25, 1989
11. Philbin DM, Rosow CE, Schneider RC, et al: Fentanyl and sufentanil anesthesia revisited: how much is enough? Anesthesiology 73:5–11, 1990
12. Reves JG, Karp RB, Buttner EE, et al: Neuronal and adrenomedullary catecholamine release in response to cardiopulmonary bypass in man. Circulation 66:49–55, 1982
13. Roberts AJ, Niarchos AP, Subramaniam VA, et al: Systemic hypertension associated with coronary artery bypass surgery: Predisposing factors, hemodynamic characteristics, humoral profile, and treatment. J Thorac Cardiovasc Surg 74:846–859, 1977
14. Liu S, Carpenter RL, Neal JM: Epidural anesthesia and analgesia: Their role in postoperative outcome (review article). Anesthesiology 82:1474–1506, 1995
15. Feigl EO: Coronary physiology (review article). Physiol Rev 63:1–205, 1983
16. Lee DD, Kimura S, DeQuattro V: Noradrenergic activity and silent ischaemia in hypertensive patients with stable angina: Effect of metoprolol. Lancet 1:403–406, 1989
17. Vanhoutte PM, Shimokawa H: Endothelium-derived relaxing factor and coronary vasospasm. Circulation 80:1–9, 1989
18. Blomberg S, Emanuelsson H, Kvist H, et al: Effects of thoracic

epidural anesthesia on coronary arteries and arterioles in patients with coronary artery disease. Anesthesiology 73:840–847, 1990

19. Blomberg S, Emanuelsson H, Ricksten S-E: Thoracic epidural anesthesia and central hemodynamics in patients with unstable angina pectoris. Anesth Analg 69:558–562, 1989
20. Heusch G, Deussen A, Thamer V: Cardiac sympathetic nerve activity and progressive vasoconstriction distal to coronary stenosis: Feed-back aggravation of myocardial ischemia. J Auton Nerv Syst 13:311–326, 1985
21. Heusch G, Deussen A: The effects of cardiac sympathetic nerve stimulation on perfusion of stenotic coronary arteries in the dog. Circ Res 53:8–15, 1983
22. Uchida Y, Murao S: Excitation of afferent cardiac sympathetic nerve fibers during coronary occulsion. Am J Physiol 226:1094–1099, 1974
23. Mangano DT: Perioperative cardiac morbidity (review article). Anesthesiology 72: 153–184, 1990
24. Birkett DA, Apthorp GH, Chamberlain DA, et al: Bilateral upper thoracic sympathectomy in angina pectoris: Results in 52 cases. Br Med J 2:187–190, 1965
25. Kock M, Blomberg S, Emanuelsson H, et al: Thoracic epidural anesthesia improves global and regional left ventricular function during stress-induced myocardial ischemia in patients with coronary artery disease. Anesth Analg 71:625–630, 1990
26. Blomberg SG: Long-term home self-treatment with high thoracic epidural anesthesia in patients with severe coronary artery disease. Anesth Analg 79:413–421, 1994
27. Blomberg S, Curelaru I, Emanuelsson H, et al: Thoracic epidural anesthesia in patients with unstable angina pectoris. Eur Heart J 10:437–444, 1989
28. Davis RF, DeBoer LWV, Maroko PR: Thoracic epidural anesthesia reduces myocardial infarct size after coronary occlusion in dogs. Anesth Analg 65:711–717, 1986
29. Klassen GA, Bramwell RS, Bromage PR, Zborowska-Slvis DT: Effect of acute sympathectomy by epidural anesthesia on the canine coronary circulation. Anesthesiology 52:8–15, 1980
30. Alhashemi JA, Sharpe MD, Harris CL, et al: Effect of subarachnoid morphine administration on extubation time after coronary artery bypass graft surgery. J Cardiothorac Vasc Anesth 14:639–644, 2000
31. Latham P, Zarate E, White PF, et al: Fast-track cardiac anesthesia: a comparison of remifentanil plus intrathecal morphine with sufentanil in a desflurane-based anesthetic. J Cardiothorac Vasc Anesth 14:645–651, 2000
32. Zarate E, Latham P, White PF, et al: Fast-track cardiac anesthesia: Use of remifentanil combined with intrathecal morphine as an al-

ternative to sufentanil during desflurane anesthesia. Anesth Analg 91:283–287, 2000

33. Bowler I, Djaiani G, Hall J, et al: Intravenous remifentanil combined with intrathecal morphine decreases extubation times after elective coronary artery bypass graft (CABG) surgery (abstract). Anesth Analg 90:S33, 2000

34. Lee TWR, Jacobsohn E, Maniate JM, et al: High spinal anesthesia in cardiac surgery: Effects on hemodynamics, perioperative stress response, and atrial b-receptor function (abstract). Anesth Analg 90:SCA90, 2000

35. Peterson KL, DeCampli WM, Pike NA, et al: A report of two hundred twenty cases of regional anesthesia in pediatric cardiac surgery. Anesth Analg 90:1014–1019, 2000

36. Hammer GB, Ngo K, Macario A: A retrospective examination of regional plus general anesthesia in children undergoing open heart surgery. Anesth Analg 90:1020–1024, 2000

37. Djaiani G, Bowler I, Hall J, et al: A combination of remifentanil and intrathecal morphine improves pulmonary function following CABG surgery (abstract). Anesth Analg 90:SCA64, 2000

38. Chaney MA, Nikolov MP, Blakeman BP, Bakhos M: Intrathecal morphine for coronary artery bypass graft procedure and early extubation revisited. J Cardiothorac Vasc Anesth 13:574–578, 1999

39. Shroff A, Rooke GA, Bishop MJ: Effects of intrathecal opioid on extubation time, analgesia, and intensive care unit stay following coronary artery bypass grafting. J Clin Anesth 9:415–419, 1997

40. Chaney MA, Furry PA, Fluder EM, Slogoff S: Intrathecal morphine for coronary artery bypass grafting and early extubation. Anesth Analg 84:241–248, 1997

41. Chaney MA, Smith KR, Barclay JC, Slogoff S: Large-dose intrathecal morphine for coronary artery bypass grafting. Anesth Analg 83:215–222, 1996

42. Kowalewski R, MacAdams C, Froelich J, et al: Anesthesia supplemented with subarachnoid bupivacaine and morphine for coronary artery bypass surgery in a child with Kawasaki disease (case report). J Cardiothorac Vasc Anesth 10:243–246, 1996

43. Taylor A, Healy M, McCarroll M, Moriarty DC: Intrathecal morphine: One year's experience in cardiac surgical patients. J Cardiothorac Vasc Anesth 10:225–228, 1996

44. Kowalewski RJ, MacAdams CL, Eagle CJ, et al: Anaesthesia for coronary artery bypass surgery supplemented with subarachnoid bupivacaine and morphine: a report of 18 cases. Can J Anaesth 41:1189–1195, 1994

45. Swenson JD, Hullander RM, Wingler K, Leivers D: Early extuba-

tion after cardiac surgery using combined intrathecal sufentanil and morphine. J Cardiothorac Vasc Anesth 8:509–514, 1994

46. Shroff AB, Bishop MJ: Intrathecal morphine analgesia speeds extubation and shortens ICU stay following coronary artery bypass grafting (CABG) (abstract). Anesthesiology 81:A129, 1994

47. Fitzpatrick GJ, Moriarty DC: Intrathecal morphine in the management of pain following cardiac surgery: A comparison with morphine i.v. Br J Anaesth 60:639–644, 1988

48. Vanstrum GS, Bjornson KM, Ilko R: Postoperative effects of intrathecal morphine in coronary artery bypass surgery. Anesth Analg 67:261–267,1988

49. Casey WF, Wynands JE, Ralley FE, et al: The role of intrathecal morphine in the anesthetic management of patients undergoing coronary artery bypass surgery. J Cardiothorac Anesth 1:510–516, 1987

50. Cheun JK: Intraspinal narcotic anesthesia in open heart surgery. J Kor Med Sci 2:225–229, 1987

51. Aun C, Thomas D, St. John-Jones L, et al: Intrathecal morphine in cardiac surgery. Eur J Anaesthesiol 2:419–426, 1985

52. Vincenty C, Malone B, Mathru M, Venus B: Comparison of intrathecal and intravenous morphine in post coronary bypass surgery (abstract). Crit Care Med 13:308, 1985

53. Jones SEF, Beasley JM, Macfarlane DWR, et al: Intrathecal morphine for postoperative pain relief in children. Br J Anaesth 56:137–140, 1984

54. Mathews ET, Abrams LD: Intrathecal morphine in open heart surgery (correspondence). Lancet 2:543, 1980

55. Chaney MA: Side effects of intrathecal and epidural opioids (review article). Can J Anaesth 42:891–903, 1995

56. Wang JK, Nauss LA, Thomas JE: Pain relief by intrathecally applied morphine in man. Anesthesiology 50:149–151, 1979

57. Behar M, Magora F, Oslhwang D, Davidson JT: Epidural morphine in treatment of pain. Lancet 1:527–528, 1979

58. Glynn CJ, Mather LE, Cousins MJ, et al: Spinal narcotics and respiratory depression (correspondence). Lancet 2:356–357, 1979

59. Liolios A, Anderson FH: Selective spinal analgesia (correspondence). Lancet 2:357, 1979

60. Scott DB, McClure J: Selective epidural analgesia (correspondence). Lancet 1:1410–1411, 1979

61. Shook JE, Watkins WD, Camporesi EM: Differential roles of opioid receptors in respiration, respiratory disease, and opiate-induced respiratory depression. Am Rev Respir Dis 142:895–909, 1990

62. Sivarajan M, Amory DW, Lindbloom LE, Schwettmann RS: Systemic and regional blood-flow changes during spinal anesthesia in the rhesus monkey. Anesthesiology 43:78–88, 1975

63. Hackel DB, Sancetta SM, Kleinerman J: Effect of hypotension due

to spinal anesthesia on coronary blood flow and myocardial metabolism in man. Circulation 13:92–97, 1956

64. Reiz S, Nath S, Rais O: Effects of thoracic epidural block and prenalterol on coronary vascular resistance and myocardial metabolism in patients with coronary artery disease. Acta Anaesthesiol Scand 24:11–6, 1980

65. DiNardo JA, Bert A, Schwartz MJ, et al: Effects of vasoactive drugs on flows through left internal mammary artery and saphenous vein grafts in man. J Thorac Cardiovasc Surg 102:730–735, 1991

66. Heusch G: α-Adrenergic mechanisms in myocardial ischemia. Circulation 81:1–13, 1990

67. Vandermeulen EP, Van Aken H, Vermylen J: Anticoagulants and spinal-epidural anesthesia. Anesth Analg 79:1165–1177, 1994

68. Markham JW, Lynge HN, Stahlman GEB: The syndrome of spontaneous spinal epidural hematoma: Report of three cases. J Neurosurg 26:334–342, 1967

69. Waldman SD, Feldstein GS, Waldman HJ, et al: Caudal administration of morphine sulfate in anticoagulated and thrombocytopenic patients. Anesth Analg 66:267–268, 1987

70. Odoom JA, Sih IL: Epidural analgesia and anticoagulant therapy: Experience with one thousand cases of continuous epidurals. Anaesthesia 38:254–259, 1983

71. Owens EL, Kasten GW, Hessel EA: Spinal subarachnoid hematoma after lumbar puncture and heparinization: A case report, review of the literature, and discussion of anesthetic implications. Anesth Analg 65:1201–1207, 1986

72. Brem SS, Hafler DA, Van Uitert RL, et al: Spinal subarachnoid hematoma: A hazard of lumbar puncture resulting in reversible paraplegia. N Engl J Med 303:1020–1021, 1981

73. Ruff RL, Dougherty JH: Complications of lumbar puncture followed by anticoagulation. Stroke 12:879–881, 1981

74. Varkey GP, Brindle GF: Peridural anaesthesia and anticoagulant therapy. Can Anaesth Soc J 21:106–109, 1974

75. Baron HC, LaRaja RD, Rossi G, Atkinson D: Continuous epidural analgesia in the heparinized vascular surgical patient: A retrospective review of 912 patients. J Vasc Surg 6:144–146, 1987

76. Rao TLK, El-Etr AA: Anticoagulation following placement of epidural and subarachnoid catheters: an evaluation of neurologic sequelae. Anesthesiology 55:618–620, 1981

77. Ho AMH, Chung DC, Joynt GM: Neuraxial blockade and hematoma in cardiac surgery: Estimating the risk of a rare adverse event that has not (yet) occurred. Chest 117:551–555, 2000

78. Goldstein S, Dean D, Kim SJ, et al: A survey of spinal and epidural techniques in adult cardiac surgery. J Cardiothorac Vasc Anesth 15:158–168, 2001

Mark A. Chaney, M.D.

4 Epidural Techniques for Adult Cardiac Surgery

INTRODUCTION

Inadequate analgesia and/or an uninhibited stress response during the postoperative period may lead to many adverse hemodynamic, metabolic, immunologic, and hemostatic alterations (1–3). Aggressive control of postoperative pain with regional anesthesia and analgesia, associated with an attenuated stress response, may decrease morbidity and mortality in high-risk patients after noncardiac surgery (4, 5). Aggressive control of postoperative pain with intravenous (IV) analgesics, associated with an attenuated stress response in patients after cardiac surgery, may also decrease morbidity and mortality (6, 7). The perioperative use of intrathecal (IT) or epidural (EPI) anesthesia and analgesia in patients undergoing cardiac surgery may beneficially affect outcome by producing intense postoperative analgesia, stress-response attenuation, and thoracic cardiac sympathectomy (8). However, the technique can be associated with undesirable drug effects that may possibly increase morbidity, and it entails an increased risk of hematoma formation (8). This chapter summarizes the risks and benefits associated with the application of EPI anesthesia and analgesia in patients undergoing cardiac surgery and suggests future directions for investigation.

Regional Anesthesia for Cardiothoracic Surgery, edited by Mark Chaney, Lippincott Williams & Wilkins, Baltimore © 2002.

POTENTIAL BENEFITS

In patients undergoing cardiac surgery, perioperative myocardial ischemia (diagnosed by electrocardiography and/or transesophageal echocardiography) is most commonly observed during the immediate postoperative period (25%–38% incidence) and is related to outcome (9, 10).
Intraoperatively, initiation of cardiopulmonary bypass (CPB) causes significant increases in stress-response hormones (nonepinephrine, epinephrine, etc.) that persist into the immediate postoperative period and may
contribute to myocardial ischemia observed during this time (11–13). Furthermore, postoperative myocardial ischemia may be aggravated by cardiac sympathetic nerve activation, which disrupts the balance between
coronary blood flow and myocardial oxygen demand (14). During the pivotal immediate postoperative period after cardiac surgery, the major potential benefits offered by EPI anesthesia and analgesia are intense analgesia, stress-response attenuation, and thoracic cardiac sympathectomy.

Intense Postoperative Analgesia

Aggressive control of postoperative pain in patients after cardiac surgery may beneficially affect outcome. In adults undergoing coronary
artery bypass grafting (CABG), intense analgesia (continuous IV sufentanil infusion) during the immediate postoperative period (first 18
hours) decreases the incidence and severity of myocardial ischemia as
diagnosed by the electrocardiography (6). In neonates undergoing cardiac surgery, intense analgesia (continuous IV fentanyl or sufentanil infusion) during the immediate postoperative period (first 24 hours) decreases morbidity and mortality (7). Unfortunately, aggressive control
of pain with IV opioids in this manner does not allow tracheal extubation to occur in the immediate postoperative period. EPI anesthesia and
analgesia is an attractive alternative to IV opioids in this setting for its
potential to produce intense analgesia yet still allow extubation to occur
in the immediate postoperative period.

Stress Response Attenuation

An uninhibited stress response during the postoperative period may
lead to many adverse hemodynamic (tachycardia, hypertension, vasoconstriction), metabolic (increased catabolism), immunologic (impaired
immune response), and hemostatic (platelet activation) alterations (1–3).
EPI anesthesia and analgesia (with local anesthetics or opioids) can effectively inhibit the stress response associated with surgical procedures

(14). Local anesthetics appear to possess greater efficacy than opioids in stress-response attenuation, perhaps because of their unique mechanism of action (14). Although still a matter of some debate, stress-response attenuation with EPI local anesthetics and/or opioids in high-risk patients after major noncardiac surgery may decrease morbidity and mortality (4, 5, 14). In patients undergoing cardiac surgery, initiation of CPB causes significant increases in stress-response hormones that persist into the immediate postoperative period (11–13). Attenuation of this component of the stress response with IV opioids may also decrease morbidity and mortality (6, 7). Unfortunately, stress-response attenuation in patients undergoing cardiac surgery with IV opioids in this manner does not allow extubation to occur in the immediate postoperative period. EPI anesthesia and analgesia (particularly with local anesthetics) is an attractive alternative to IV opioids in this setting for its potential to attenuate the stress response yet still allow extubation to occur in the immediate postoperative period.

Thoracic Cardiac Sympathectomy

The myocardium and coronary vasculature are densely innervated by sympathetic nerve fibers that arise from T1 to T5 and profoundly influence total coronary blood flow and distribution (15). Cardiac sympathetic nerve activation initiates coronary artery vasoconstriction (16) and paradoxical vasoconstriction in response to intrinsic vasodilators (17). In patients with coronary artery disease, cardiac sympathetic nerve activation disrupts the normal matching of coronary blood flow and myocardial oxygen demand (18, 19). Animal models show an intense poststenotic vasoconstrictive mechanism mediated by cardiac sympathetic nerve activation that attenuates local metabolic vasodilation in response to myocardial ischemia (20, 21). Furthermore, myocardial ischemia initiates a cardiocardiac reflex mediated by sympathetic nerve fibers, which augments the ischemic process (22). Cardiac sympathetic nerve activation likely plays a central role in initiating postoperative myocardial ischemia by decreasing the myocardial oxygen supply via the mechanisms listed above (14, 23).

Thoracic EPI anesthesia with local anesthetics effectively blocks cardiac sympathetic nerve afferent and efferent fibers (14). Opioids, which are administered similarly, are unable to effectively block cardiac sympathetic nerve activity (14). Patients with symptomatic coronary artery disease benefit from cardiac sympathectomy, and the application of thoracic sympathetic blockade in the management of angina pectoris was described as early as 1965 (24). Thoracic EPI anesthesia with local anesthetics increases the diameter of stenotic epicardial coronary artery segments without causing dilation of coronary arterioles (18), decreases determinants of myocardial oxygen demand (19), improves left ventricular function (25), and decreases anginal symptoms (26, 27). Furthermore, cardiac sympathectomy increases the endocardial to epicardial blood flow ratio (28, 29), beneficially affects collateral blood flow during myocardial ischemia (29), decreases poststenotic vasoconstriction (21), and attenuates the myocardial ischemia-induced cardiocardiac reflex (21). In an animal model, thoracic EPI anesthesia with local anesthetics decreases myocardial infarct size after coronary artery occlusion (28). Of note, these beneficial effects are not caused by systemic absorption of the local anesthetic (28). In short, thoracic EPI anesthesia with local anesthetics may benefit patients undergoing cardiac surgery by effectively blocking cardiac sympathetic nerve activity and improving the myocardial oxygen supply–demand balance.

CLINICAL UTILIZATION OF EPIDURAL TECHNIQUES

Table 4–1 summarizes the clinical investigations detailing application of EPI anesthesia and analgesia to patients undergoing cardiac surgery (30–53). Application of EPI anesthesia and analgesia to patients undergoing cardiac surgery was initially reported by Hoar et al. in 1976 (53). They described the intraoperative insertion of thoracic EPI catheters in 12 patients after CABG. The catheters were injected with lidocaine and bupivacaine during the postoperative period to promote analgesia and control hypertension (53). The 1987 article by El-Baz and Goldin (51) was the first to report the insertion of thoracic EPI catheters in patients prior to initiation of cardiac surgery. Others have subsequently applied EPI anesthesia and analgesia to patients undergoing cardiac surgery (Table 4–1). Most have used EPI local anesthetics in hopes of providing stress-response attenuation and/or thoracic cardiac sympathectomy. Some have used EPI opioids to provide intraoperative and/or postoperative analgesia.

EPI anesthesia and analgesia with local anesthetics and/or opioids induce significant postoperative analgesia in patients after cardiac surgery. Patients randomized to receive a continuous thoracic EPI morphine infusion (0.1 mg/h) after cardiac surgery required significantly less supplemental IV morphine than patients without EPI catheters (5 vs 18 mg/day per patient, respectively) during the initial 3 postoperative days (51). When compared to patients receiving only general anesthesia, significantly less numbers of patients randomized to receive a continuous thoracic EPI bupivacaine infusion after cardiac surgery required supplemental IV analgesics during the immediate postoperative

TABLE 4–1. Reports Of Epidural Anesthesia And Analgesia For Cardiac Surgery

Author (reference)	Year	Study Design	Total Patients	Drugs: Dose	Intraoperative Management	Remarks
Jideus et al. (30)	2001	Prospective, randomized	41	Bupivacaine: bolus plus infusion Sufentanil: infusion	Not standardized	Stress response attenuation Thoracic cardiac sympathectomy
Scott et al. (31)	2001	Prospective, randomized	206	Bupivacaine: bolus plus infusion Clonidine: infusion	Standardized	Decreased postoperative arrhythmias Improved postoperative pulmonary function Decreased postoperative renal failure Decreased postoperative confusion
Warters et al. (32)+	2000	Retrospective	278	Not specified	Not standardized	No hematoma formation
Loick et al. (33)	1999	Prospective, randomized	25	Bupivacaine: bolus plus infusion Sufentanil: bolus plus infusion	Standardized	Stress response attenuation Thoracic cardiac sympathectomy Facilitated early extubation
Tenling et al. (34)	1999	Prospective, randomized	14	Bupivacaine: bolus plus Infusion	Not standardized	Reliable postoperative analgesia Facilitated early extubation
Sanchez and Nygard (35)	1998	Prospective, observational	571	Bupivacaine: boluses	Not standardized	No hematoma formation
Loick et al. (36)*	1998	Prospective, randomized	25	Not specified	Not specified	Reliable postoperative analgesia Stress response attenuation Thoracic cardiac sympathectomy Facilitated early extubation *(continued)*

TABLE 4–1. Reports Of Epidural Anesthesia And Analgesia For Cardiac Surgery (*Continued*)

Author (reference)	Year	Study Design	Total Patients	Drugs: Dose	Intraoperative Management	Remarks
Warters et al. (37)*	1998	Retrospective	278	Not specified	Not standardized	No hematoma formation
Shayevitz et al. (38)	1996	Retrospective	54	Morphine: bolus plus infusion	Not standardized	Reliable postoperative analgesia Facilitated early extubation
Frank et al. (39)*	1995	Retrospective	29	Morphine: bolus and / or infusion	Not standardized	Facilitated early extubation
Moore et al (40)	1995	Prospective, randomized	17	Bupivacaine: bolus plus infusion	Standardized	Stress response attenuation Possible thoracic cardiac sympathectomy
Stenseth et al. (41)	1995	Prospective, randomized	30	Bupivacaine: bolus plus Infusion	Standardized	Thoracic cardiac sympathectomy
Kirno et al. (42)	1994	Prospective, randomized	20	Mepivacaine: bolus	Standardized	Stress response attenuation Thoracic cardiac sympathectomy
Stenseth et al. (43, 44)	1994	Prospective, randomized	30	Bupivacaine: bolus plus infusion	Standardized	Stress response attenuation Possible thoracic cardiac sympathectomy (*continued*)

TABLE 4–1. Reports Of Epidural Anesthesia And Analgesia For Cardiac Surgery (*Continued*)

Author (reference)	Year	Study Design	Total Patients	Drugs: Dose	Intraoperative Management	Remarks
Shapiro et al. (45)*	1994	Prospective, observational	41	Morphine: bolus	Not standardized	Reliable postoperative analgesia
Liem et al. (46–48)	1992	Prospective, randomized	54	Bupivacaine: bolus plus infusion Sufentanil: bolus plus infusion	Not standardized	Reliable postoperative analgesia Stress response attenuation Possible thoracic cardiac sympathectomy
Rosen and Rosen (49)	1989	Prospective, randomized	32	Morphine: bolus	Not standardized	Reliable postoperative analgesia Facilitated early extubation
Joachimsson et al. (50)	1989	Observational	28	Bupivacaine: boluses	Not standardized	Reliable postoperative analgesia
El-Baz and Goldin (51)	1987	Prospective, randomized	60	Morphine: infusion	Standardized	Reliable postoperative analgesia Stress response attenuation Facilitated early extubation
Robinson et al. (52)	1986	Prospective, observational	10	Meperidine: bolus	Standardized	Reliable postoperative analgesia
Hoar et al. (53)	1976	Prospective, observational	12	Lidocaine: boluses Bupivacaine: boluses	Not standardized	Reliable postoperative analgesia Possible stress response attenuation

* = Abstract
+ = Correspondence

period (34). Children (age 2–12 years) randomized to receive caudal EPI morphine (75 mcg/kg) intraoperatively after cardiac surgery required significantly less supplemental IV morphine than patients who did not receive EPI morphine (0.32 vs 0.71 mg/kg, respectively) during the initial 24 postoperative hours (49). Many other studies further attest to the ability of EPI anesthesia and analgesia with local anesthetics and/or opioids to induce substantial postoperative analgesia in patients after cardiac surgery (36, 38, 45, 47, 50, 52, 53).

EPI anesthesia with local anesthetics significantly attenuates the stress response in patients undergoing cardiac surgery. Patients randomized to receive intermittent boluses of thoracic EPI bupivacaine intraoperatively followed by continuous infusion postoperatively exhibited significantly decreased blood levels of norepinephrine and epinephrine perioperatively when compared with patients managed similarly without EPI catheters (44). Furthermore, increased blood catecholamine levels in these patients were associated with increased systemic vascular resistance (44). Patients randomized to receive a continuous thoracic EPI bupivacaine infusion perioperatively exhibited significantly decreased blood levels of norepinephrine and cortisol perioperatively when compared with patients managed similarly without EPI catheters (40). Patients randomized to receive a continuous thoracic EPI bupivacaine and sufentanil infusion perioperatively exhibited significantly decreased blood levels of norepinephrine after sternotomy when compared with patients managed similarly without EPI catheters (48).

Two more recently performed clinical investigations have again revealed the ability of EPI anesthesia with local anesthetics to significantly attenuate the stress response in patients undergoing cardiac surgery (30, 33). Loick et al. demonstrated that patients randomized to receive thoracic EPI bupivacaine and sufentanil exhibited significantly lower perioperative plasma epinephrine levels when compared to control patients (33). Jideus et al. demonstrated that patients randomized to receive thoracic EPI bupivacaine and sufentanil exhibited significantly lower perioperative plasma levels of norepinephrine, epinephrine, and neuropeptide Y when compared to control patients (30). Other studies further attest to the ability of EPI anesthesia with local anesthetics to promote perioperative hemodynamic stability in patients undergoing cardiac surgery, which suggests stress response attenuation (42, 43, 46, 53).

One study indicates that EPI analgesia with opioids significantly attenuates the stress response in patients undergoing cardiac surgery (51). Patients randomized to receive a continuous thoracic EPI morphine infusion postoperatively exhibited significantly decreased blood levels of cortisol and β-endorphin postoperatively when compared with patients managed similarly without EPI catheters (51).

Three provocative studies demonstrate the ability of EPI anesthesia to induce significant thoracic cardiac sympathectomy in patients undergoing cardiac surgery (33, 41, 42). Kirno et al. in 1994 studied patients undergoing CABG who were evaluated with catheters that had been placed in the coronary sinus under fluoroscopic guidance and continuous pressure monitoring prior to induction of anesthesia (42). Intraoperative anesthetic management was standardized, and all patients received a continuous IV infusion of tritiated norepinephrine (42). To assess cardiac sympathetic activity, blood samples were obtained from the coronary sinus and radial artery, and the rate of norepinephrine spillover from the heart was calculated according to the Fick principle (42). Patients randomized to receive a single bolus of thoracic EPI mepivacaine immediately after the induction of anesthesia exhibited significantly decreased cardiac norepinephrine spillover after sternotomy when compared with patients managed similarly without EPI catheters (42). Furthermore, 20% of patients managed without EPI catheters exhibited electrocardiographic evidence of myocardial ischemia after sternotomy, whereas no patient managed with an EPI catheter exhibited myocardial ischemia during this time (42).

Stenseth et al. in 1995 studied patients undergoing CABG who were evaluated with reverse thermodilution catheters that had been placed in the mid-coronary sinus under fluoroscopic guidance prior to the induction of anesthesia (41). Intraoperative anesthetic management was standardized. Coronary sinus blood blow was measured by a constant infusion technique, and coronary vascular resistance was calculated utilizing coronary perfusion pressure (arterial diastolic pressure minus pulmonary capillary wedge pressure) and coronary sinus blood flow (41). Patients who had been randomized to receive intermittent boluses of thoracic EPI bupivacaine intraoperatively followed by continuous infusion postoperatively exhibited significant decreases in coronary vascular resistance post-CPB when compared with pre-CPB values, whereas patients managed similarly without EPI catheters exhibited significant increases in coronary vascular resistance post-CPB (41).

Finally, Loick et al. in 1999 studied patients undergoing CABG who were evaluated for perioperative myocardial ischemia via plasma levels of myocardial-specific contractile protein troponin T (and other cardiac enzymes) and electrocardiographic monitoring (33). Intraoperative anesthetic management was standardized. Patients who had been randomized to receive intermittent boluses of thoracic EPI bupivacaine and sufentanil intraoperatively followed by continuous infusion postoperatively exhibited significantly lower postoperative troponin T levels and substantially less postoperative electrocardiographic evidence of myocardial ischemia when compared to control patients not receiving thoracic EPI bupivacaine and sufentanil (33).

Perioperative cardiac sympathectomy induced via thoracic EPI anesthesia with local anesthetics may benefit patients undergoing cardiac surgery by increasing the myocardial oxygen supply (18, 28, 29). However, such a cardiac sympathectomy offers additional benefits to patients undergoing cardiac surgery. Multiple studied demonstrate that EPI anesthesia with local anesthetics significantly decreases heart rate before and after CPB (30, 33, 40, 46, 47) and significantly decreases the need to administer β-blockers after CPB (43). Multiple studies also demonstrate that EPI anesthesia with local anesthetics significantly decreases systemic vascular resistance before and after CPB (42, 44, 47, 50). Furthermore, patients undergoing cardiac surgery who received thoracic EPI anesthesia with local anesthetics not only exhibited significant decreases in postoperative heart rate and systemic vascular resistance but also exhibited significant decreases in postoperative electrocardiographic evidence of myocardial ischemia when compared with patients managed similarly without EPI catheters (47).

In summary, administration of EPI opioids or local anesthetics to patients before and/or after CPB initiates reliable postoperative analgesia after cardiac surgery. Administration of EPI local anesthetics (not opioids) can both reliably attenuate the stress response associated with CPB that persists during the immediate postoperative period and induce thoracic cardiac sympathectomy.

Clinical Outcome

The vast majority of reports detailing use of EPI anesthesia and analgesia for cardiac surgery involve small numbers of patients and few are well designed (Table 4–1). None exist that are prospective, randomized, blind, and placebo-controlled (the performance of a sham epidural insertion is considered by most to be unethical given the risk of epidural hematoma formation). The few investigations involving fairly large numbers of patients exist in abstract form (37), were published as correspondence (32), or were very limited in scope (35). Furthermore, only a few investigations use clinical outcome as a primary end point. Thus, there are clear deficiencies in the literature that prohibit definitive analysis of the risk-benefit ratio of EPI anesthesia and analgesia for cardiac surgery.

In an attempt to fill this void, Scott et al. recently published a fairly large (420 total patients) prospective, randomized study that evaluated the effect of thoracic EPI anesthesia and analgesia on clinical outcome in patients undergoing CABG (31). Two hundred six patients who received perioperative thoracic EPI supplementation (bupivacaine and clonidine continuous infusion) to general anesthesia were compared to 202 patients receiving general anesthesia alone (31). Intraoperative anesthetic management was standardized. Interestingly, they found that patients receiving thoracic EPI supplementation exhibited significantly fewer supraventricular arrhythmias ($p = 0.0012$), improved maximal inspiratory lung volumes ($p < 0.0001$), fewer lower respiratory tract infections ($p = 0.0007$), less acute confusion ($p = 0.031$), and less renal failure ($p = 0.016$) when compared to patients receiving general anesthesia alone (31). Also, postoperative extubation time was significantly decreased ($p < 0.0001$) in the thoracic EPI group when compared to the general anesthesia group (31). Many other studies further attest to the ability of EPI anesthesia to facilitate early extubation in patients during the immediate postoperative period following cardiac surgery (33, 34, 36, 38, 39, 49, 51). The results of the investigation by Scott et al. regarding clinical outcome are certainly intriguing and the authors justifiably conclude that "these findings merit a further multicenter prospective clinical trial that should focus on underlying mechanisms, long-term follow-up and outcome, and cost-effectiveness and implications for health resource consumption for the procedure" (31).

UNDESIRABLE DRUG EFFECTS

Opioids

Although many have been described, the four clinically relevant undesirable drug effects of EPI opioids are pruritus, nausea and vomiting, urinary retention, and respiratory depression (54). After administration of EPI opioids, the most common side effect is pruritus. The incidence varies widely, from 0% to 100%, and is often identified only after direct questioning of patients. Severe pruritus is rare, occurring in only approximately 1% of patients. The incidence of nausea and vomiting is approximately 30%. The incidence of urinary retention varies widely, from 0% to 80%, and occurs most frequently in young male patients. When EPI opioids are used in patients undergoing cardiac surgery, the incidence of pruritus, nausea and vomiting, and urinary pretension is similar to that described above (38, 49, 51).

The most important undesirable drug effect of EPI opioids is respiratory depression. Only 4 months after the initial use of IT (55) and EPI (56) opioids in humans in 1979, life-threatening respiratory depression was reported (57–59). The incidence of respiratory depression that requires intervention after conventional doses of EPI opioids is approximately 1%, the same as that after conventional doses of intramuscular and IV opioids. Early respiratory depression occurs within minutes of opioid injection and is associated with administration of EPI fentanyl or sufentanil. Delayed respiratory depression occurs hours after opioid injection and is associated with administration of EPI morphine. Delayed respiratory depression results from cephalad migration of morphine in cerebrospinal fluid and the subsequent stimulation of opioid receptors located in the ventral medulla (60). Factors that increase the risk of respiratory depression include large and/or repeated doses of opioids, intrathecal utilization, advanced age, and concomitant use of IV sedatives (54). Unlike some investigations involving IT morphine, no investigations involving use of EPI opioids in patients undergoing cardiac surgery describe prolonged postoperative respiratory depression that significantly increases extubation time (8). This is likely due to the fact that the vast majority of investigations involving EPI anesthesia and analgesia in patients undergoing cardiac surgery have focused primarily on stress response attenuation and/or thoracic cardiac sympathectomy and thus used local anesthetics (with or without dilute opioid concentrations) (8).

Local Anesthetics

The most troubling and undesirable drug effect of EPI local anesthetics is hypotension. Spinal anesthesia to upper thoracic dermatomes produces a decrease in mean arterial blood pressure that is accompanied by a parallel decrease in coronary blood flow (61, 62). Exactly what percentage of blood pressure decrease is acceptable remains speculative, especially in patients with coronary artery disease. Disturbances in myocardial oxygenation occur in patients with coronary artery disease if coronary perfusion pressure is allowed to decrease by more than 50% during induction of thoracic EPI anesthesia with local anesthetics (63). Furthermore, if alpha adrenergic agonists are used to increase blood pressure, there may be detrimental effects (vasoconstriction) on the native coronary arteries and bypass grafts (64, 65). Hypotension appears to be relatively common when EPI local anesthetics are used in the setting of cardiac surgery (40–43). Volume replacement, β-agonists, or α-agonists are required in 50% to 90% of patients (40–43), and coronary perfusion pressure may decrease after CPB (41, 43).

After EPI administration, local anesthetics can produce blood concentrations of drug that may cause detrimental cardiac electrophysiologic effects and myocardial depression (66). Myocardial depression has been detected in patients receiving thoracic EPI anesthesia with bupivacaine, an effect at least partially caused by increased blood concentrations of the drug (67). Concomitant use of β-blockers may further decrease myocardial contractility in this setting (68, 69). Patients undergoing cardiac surgery who were randomized to receive intermittent boluses of thoracic EPI bupivacaine intraoperatively followed by continuous infusion postoperatively exhibited significantly increased pulmonary capillary wedge pressures post-CPB when compared with patients managed similarly without EPI catheters (10.8 vs 6.4 mm Hg, respectively), which suggests myocardial depression (43).

RISK OF HEMATOMA FORMATION

EPI instrumentation entails risk, the most feared complication being epidural hematoma formation. The estimated incidence of hematoma formation is approximately 1:220,000 after IT injection (70). Hematoma formation is more common (approximately 1:150,000) after EPI instrumentation because larger needles are used, catheters are placed, and the venous plexus in the EPI space is prominent (70). Furthermore, hematoma formation does not occur exclusively during EPI catheter insertion; almost half of all cases develop after catheter removal (70).

Although spontaneous hematomas can occur in the absence of EPI instrumentation (71), most occur when EPI instrumentation is performed in a patient with a coagulopathy (from any cause) or when instrumentation is difficult or traumatic (70). Paradoxically, IT or EPI instrumentation has been performed safely in patients with known coagulapathy (72, 73). Of 1000 epidural catheterizations performed in 950 patients receiving oral anticoagulants at time of catheter insertion, none developed signs or symptoms of hematoma formation (73). Of 336 epidural injections performed in 36 patients with chronic cancer pain either fully anticoagulated (oral anticoagulants or IV heparin) or profoundly thrombocytopenic (platelet count <50,000/mm^3) at the time of instrumentation, none developed signs or symptoms of hematoma formation (72).

Risk is increased when EPI instrumentation is performed prior to systemic heparinization, and hematoma formation has occurred in patients when diagnostic or therapeutic lumbar puncture has been followed by systemic heparinization (74–77). When lumbar puncture is followed by systemic heparinization, concurrent use of aspirin, difficult or traumatic instrumentation, and administration of IV heparin within one hour of instrumentation increases the risk of hematoma formation (76). However, by observing certain precautions, EPI instrumentation can be performed safely in patients who will subsequently receive IV heparin (78, 79). By delaying surgery 24 hours in the event of a traumatic tap, by delaying heparinization 60 minutes after catheter insertion, and by maintaining tight perioperative control of anticoagulation, more than 4,000 IT or EPI catheterizations were performed safely in patients undergoing peripheral vascular surgery who received IV heparin after catheter insertion (79). A retrospective review involving 912 patients further indicates that EPI catheterization prior to systematic heparinization for peripheral vascular surgery is safe (78). However, the magnitude of anticoagulation in these two studies, activated partial thromboplastin time approximately 100 seconds (78) and activated clotting time approximately twice the baseline value (79), involving patients undergoing peripheral vascular surgery was significantly less than the degree of anticoagulation required in patients subjected to CPB.

Most studies investigating the use of EPI anesthesia and analgesia in patients undergoing cardiac surgery include precautions to decrease risk of hematoma formation. Some used the technique only after the demonstration of laboratory evidence of normal coagulation parameters, delayed surgery 24 hours in the event of traumatic tap, or required that the time from instrumentation to systemic heparinization exceed 60 minutes. While most studied investigating use of EPI anesthesia and analgesia in patients undergoing cardiac surgery insert catheters the day before scheduled surgery, recent investigators have performed instrumentation on the same day of surgery (31, 32, 37). Institutional practice (same-day admit surgery) may eliminate the option of EPI catheter insertion on the day before scheduled surgery. An alternative is to perform EPI instrumentation postoperatively (prior to or after extubation), after the demonstration via laboratory evidence of normal coagulation parameters (49, 52, 53).

Although hematoma formation has never been reported in a patient receiving EPI instrumentation prior to systemic heparinization required for CPB, the risk may be as high as 0.35% (74). A recently published extensive mathematical analysis by Ho et al. of the approximately 4,583 EPI injections in patients subjected to systemic heparinization required for CPB (without a single episode of hematoma formation) reported in the literature as of the year 2000 estimated that the minimum risk of hematoma formation was 1:150,000 and the maximum risk of hematoma formation was 1:1,500 (95% confidence level) yet the maximum risk may be as high as 1:1,000 (99% confidence level) (80). Certain precautions, however, may decrease the risk (70, 74). The technique should not be used in a patient with known coagulopathy from any cause. Surgery should be delayed 24 hours in the event of a traumatic tap, and time from instrumentation to systemic heparinization should exceed 60 minutes. Additionally, heparin effect and reversal should be tightly controlled (smallest amount of heparin for the shortest duration compatible with therapeutic objectives), and patients should be closely monitored postoperatively for signs and symptoms of hematoma formation. An obvious economic disadvantage of EPI instrumentation in patients prior to cardiac surgery is the possible delay in surgery in the event of a traumatic tap.

SUMMARY AND FUTURE DIRECTIONS

The potential benefits offered by EPI anesthesia and analgesia for cardiac surgery include intense postoperative analgesia, stress response attenuation, and thoracic cardiac sympathectomy. EPI anesthesia and analgesia with opioids or local anesthetics may induce reliable postoperative analgesia in patients after cardiac surgery. Significant stress-response attenuation and thoracic cardiac sympathectomy are also reliably achieved in this setting with EPI administration of local anesthetics. The most important undesirable drug effect of opioids used in this manner is respiratory depression, which may delay postoperative tracheal extubation, whereas for local anesthetics, it is hypotension, which may decrease coronary blood flow. Although never reported in a patient receiving IT or EPI instrumentation prior to systemic heparinization required for CPB, the risk of hematoma formation is increased, and certain precautions should be observed.

It is not clear whether intense postoperative analgesia, stress response attenuation, and/or thoracic cardiac sympathectomy in patients undergoing cardiac surgery affect outcome. The vast majority of reports of EPI anesthesia and analgesia for cardiac surgery involve small numbers of patients; few are well designed, and few use clinical outcome as a primary end point. Thus, there are clear deficiencies in the literature that prohibit definitive analysis of the risk-benefit ratio of EPI anesthesia and analgesia for cardiac surgery. Despite this, a recently published anonymous survey of members of the Society of Cardiovascular Anesthesiologists by Goldstein et al. indicates that 7% of practicing anesthesiologists incorporate EPI techniques into their anesthetic management of adults undergoing cardiac surgery (81). Of these anesthesiologists, 58% practice in the United States (81). Regarding timing of instrumentation, 40% perform instrumentation before induction, 12% perform instrumentation after induction, 33% perform instrumentation at the end of surgery, and 15% perform instrumentation on the first postoperative day (81). Future directions in this fertile area should focus on development of well-designed studies with adequate numbers of patients that investigate the ability of EPI anesthesia and analgesia to affect morbidity and mortality in patients after cardiac surgery. Future studies should also investigate the potential benefit of EPI anesthesia and analgesia in patients undergoing "off-pump" CABG (without CPB). Investigators have already described use of thoracic EPI anesthesia and analgesia alone (without general endotracheal anesthesia) combined with spontaneous ventilation in patients undergoing "off-pump" CABG (82, 83). Only after such studies are performed will a definitive analysis of the risk-benefit ratio of EPI anesthesia and analgesia for cardiac surgery be possible. Until that time, the routine use of EPI anesthesia and analgesia in patients undergoing cardiac surgery will remain controversial (84–86).

References

1. Weissman C: The metabolic response to stress: an overview and update (review article). Anesthesiology 73:308–327, 1990
2. Kehlet H: Surgical stress: the role of pain and analgesia (review article). Br J Anaesth 63:189–195, 1989
3. Roizen MF: Should we all have a sympathectomy at birth? Or at least preoperatively? (editorial). Anesthesiology 68:482–484, 1988
4. Tuman KJ, McCarthy RJ, March RJ, et al: Effects of epidural anesthesia and analgesia on coagulation and outcome after major vascular surgery. Anesth Analg 73:696–704,1991
5. Yeager MP, Glass DD, Neff RK, Brinck-Johnson T: Epidural anesthesia and analgesia in high-risk surgical patients. Anesthesiology 66:729–736, 1987
6. Mangano DT, Siliciano D, Hollenberg M, et al: Postoperative myocardial ischemia: therapeutic trials using intensive analgesia following surgery. Anesthesiology 76:342–353, 1992
7. Anand KJS, Hickey PR: Halothane-morphine compared with high-dose sufentanil for anesthesia and postoperative analgesia in neonatal cardiac surgery. N Engl J Med 326:1–9, 1992
8. Chaney MA: Intrathecal and epidural anesthesia and analgesia for cardiac surgery (review article). Anesth Analg 84:1211–1221, 1997
9. Smith RC, Leung JM, Mangano DT, SPI Research Group: Postoperative myocardial ischemia in patients undergoing coronary artery bypass graft surgery. Anesthesiology 74:464–473, 1991
10. Leung JM, O'Kelly B, Browner WS, et al: Prognostic importance of postbypass regional wall-motion abnormalities in patients undergoing coronary artery bypass graft surgery. Anesthesiology 71:16–25, 1989
11. Philbin DM, Rosow CE, Schneider RC, et al: Fentanyl and sufentanil anesthesia revisited: how much is enough? Anesthesiology 73:5–11, 1990
12. Reves JG, Karp RB, Buttner EE, et al: Neuronal and adrenomedullary catecholamine release in response to cardiopulmonary bypass in man. Circulation 66:49–55, 1982
13. Roberts AJ, Niarchos AP, Subramaniam VA, et al: Systemic hypertension associated with coronary artery bypass surgery: predisposing factors, hemodynamic characteristics, humoral profile, and treatment. J Thorac Cardiovasc Surg 74:846–859, 1977
14. Liu S, Carpenter RL, Neal JM: Epidural anesthesia and analgesia:

their role in postoperative outcome (review article). Anesthesiology 82:1474–1506, 1995

15. Feigl EO: Coronary physiology (review article). Physiol Rev 63:1–205, 1983
16. Lee DD, Kimura S, DeQuattro V: Noradrenergic activity and silent ischemia in hypertensive patients with stable angina: effect of metoprolol. Lancet 1:403–406, 1989
17. Vanhoutte PM, Shimokawa H: Endothelium-derived relaxing factor and coronary vasospasm. Circulation 80:1–9, 1989
18. Blomberg S, Emanuelsson H, Kvist H, et al: Effects of thoracic epidural anesthesia on coronary arteries and arterioles in patients with coronary artery disease. Anesthesiology 73:840–847, 1990
19. Blomberg S, Emanuelsson H, Ricksten S-E: Thoracic epidural anesthesia and central hemodynamics in patients with unstable angina pectoris. Anesth Analg 69:558–562, 1989
20. Heusch G, Deussen A, Thamer V: Cardiac sympathetic nerve activity and progressive vasoconstriction distal to coronary stenosis: feed-back aggravation of myocardial ischemia. J Auton Nerv Syst 13:311–326, 1985
21. Heusch G, Deussen A: The effects of cardiac sympathetic nerve stimulation on perfusion of stenotic coronary arteries in the dog. Circ Res 53:8–15, 1983
22. Uchida Y, Murao S: Excitation of afferent cardiac sympathetic nerve fibers during coronary occlusion. Am J Physiol 226:1094–1099, 1974
23. Mangano DT: Perioperative cardiac morbidity (review article). Anesthesiology 72: 153–184, 1990
24. Birkett DA, Apthorp GH, Chamberlain DA, et al: Bilateral upper thoracic sympathectomy in angina pectoris: results in 52 cases. Br Med J 2:187–190, 1965
25. Kock M, Blomberg S, Emanuelsson H, et al: Thoracic epidural anesthesia improves global and regional left ventricular function during stress-induced myocardial ischemia in patients with coronary artery disease. Anesth Analg 71:625–630, 1990
26. Blomberg SG: Long-term home self-treatment with high thoracic epidural anesthesia in patients with severe coronary artery disease. Anesth Analg 79:413–421, 1994
27. Blomberg S, Curelaru I, Emanuelsson H, et al: Thoracic epidural anesthesia in patients with unstable angina pectoris. Eur Heart J 10:437–444, 1989
28. Davis RF, DeBoer LWV, Maroko PR: Thoracic epidural anesthesia reduces myocardial infarct size after coronary occlusion in dogs. Anesth Analg 65:711–717, 1986
29. Klassen GA, Bramwell RS, Bromage PR, Zborowska-Slvis DT:

Effect of acute sympathectomy by epidural anesthesia on the canine coronary circulation. Anesthesiology 52:8–15, 1980

30. Jideus L, Joachimsson PO, Stridsberg M, et al: Thoracic epidural anesthesia does not influence the occurrence of postoperative sustained atrial fibrillation. Ann Thorac Surg 72:65–71, 2001

31. Scott NB, Turfrey DJ, Ray DAA, et al: A prospective randomized study of the potential benefits of thoracic epidural anesthesia and analgesia in patients undergoing coronary artery bypass grafting. Anesth Analg 93:528–535, 2001

32. Warters D, Knight W, Koch SM, Luehr S: Thoracic epidurals in coronary artery bypass surgery (correspondence). Anesth Analg 90:767, 2000

33. Loick HM, Schmidt C, Van Aken H, et al: High thoracic epidural anesthesia, but not clonidine, attenuates the perioperative stress response via sympatholysis and reduces the release of troponin T in patients undergoing coronary artery bypass grafting. Anesth Analg 88:701–709, 1999

34. Tenling A, Joachimsson PO, Tyden H, et al: Thoracic epidural anesthesia as an adjunct to general anesthesia for cardiac surgery: effects on ventilation-perfusion relationships. J Cardiothorac Vasc Anesth 13:258–264, 1999

35. Sanchez R, Nygard E: Epidural anesthesia in cardiac surgery: is there an increased risk? J Cardiothorac Vasc Anesth 12:170–173, 1998

36. Loick HM, Mollhoff T, Erren M, et al: Thoracic epidural anesthesia lowers catecholamine and TNFa release after CABG in humans (abstract). Anesth Analg 86:S81, 1998

37. Warters RD, Koch SM, Luehr SL, Katz J: Thoracic epidural anesthesia in CABG surgery (abstract). Anesth Analg 86:S116, 1998

38. Shayevitz JR, Merkel S, O'Kelly SW, et al: Lumbar epidural morphine infusions for children undergoing cardiac surgery. J Cardiothorac Vasc Anesth 10: 217–224, 1996

39. Frank RS, Boltz MG, Sentivany SK, Krane EJ: Combined epidural-general anesthesia for the repair of atrial septal defects in children results in shorter ICU stays (abstract). Anesthesiology 83:A1176, 1995

40. Moore CM, Cross MH, Desborough JP, et al: Hormonal effects of thoracic extradural analgesia for cardiac surgery. Br J Anaesth 75:387–393, 1995

41. Stenseth R, Berg EM, Bjella L, et al: Effects of thoracic epidural analgesia on coronary hemodynamics and myocardial metabolism in coronary artery bypass surgery. J Cardiothorac Vasc Anesth 9: 503–509, 1995

42. Kirno K, Friberg P, Grzegorczyk A, et al: Thoracic epidural anesthesia during coronary artery bypass surgery: effects on cardiac

sympathetic activity, myocardial blood flow and metabolism, and central hemodynamics. Anesth Analg 79:1075–1081, 1994

43. Stenseth R, Bjella L, Berg M, et al: Thoracic epidural analgesia in aortocoronary bypass surgery I: hemodynamic effects. Acta Anaesthesiol Scand 38:826–833, 1994

44. Stenseth R, Bjella L, Berg M, et al: Thoracic epidural analgesia in aortocoronary bypass surgery II: effects on the endocrine metabolic response. Acta Anaesthesiol Scand 38:834–839, 1994

45. Shapiro JH, Wolman RL, Lofland GK: Epidural morphine as an adjunct for early extubation following congenital cardiac surgery (abstract). Anesth Analg 78:S385, 1994

46. Liem TH, Booij LHDJ, Hasenbos MAWM, Gielen MJM: Coronary artery bypass grafting using two different anesthetic techniques: part 1: hemodynamic results. J Cardiothorac Vasc Anesth 6:148–155, 1992

47. Liem TH, Hasenbos MAWM, Booij LHDJ, Gielen MJM: Coronary artery bypass grafting using two different anesthetic techniques: part 2: postoperative outcome. J Cardiothorac Vasc Anesth 6:156–161, 1992

48. Liem TH, Booij LHDJ, Gielen MJM, et al: Coronary artery bypass grafting using two different anesthetic techniques: part 3: adrenergic responses. J Cardiothorac Vasc Anesth 6:162–167, 1992

49. Rosen KR, Rosen DA: Caudal epidural morphine for control of pain following open heart surgery in children. Anesthesiology 70:418–421, 1989

50. Joachimsson PO, Nystrom SO, Tyden H: Early extubation after coronary artery surgery in efficiently rewarmed patients: a postoperative comparison of opioid anesthesia versus inhalational anesthesia and thoracic epidural analgesia. J Cardiothorac Anesth 3:444–454, 1989

51. El-Baz N, Goldin M: Continuous epidural infusion of morphine for pain relief after cardiac operations. J Thorac Cardiovasc Surg 93:878–883, 1987

52. Robinson RJS, Brister S, Jones E, Quigly M: Epidural meperidine analgesia after cardiac surgery. Can Anaesth Soc J 33:550–555, 1986

53. Hoar PF, Hickey RF, Ullyot DJ: Systemic hypertension following myocardial revascularization; a method of treatment using epidural anesthesia. J Thorac Cardiovasc Surg 71:859–864, 1976

54. Chaney MA: Side effects of intrathecal and epidural opioids (review article). Can J Anaesth 42:891–903, 1995

55. Wang JK, Nauss LA, Thomas JE: Pain relief by intrathecally applied morphine in man. Anesthesiology 50:149–151, 1979

56. Behar M, Magora F, Oslhwang D, Davidson JT: Epidural morphine in treatment of pain. Lancet 1:527–528, 1979

57. Glynn CJ, Mather LE, Cousins MJ, et al: Spinal narcotics and respiratory depression (correspondence). Lancet 2:356–357, 1979
58. Liolios A, Anderson FH: Selective spinal analgesia (correspondence). Lancet 2:357, 1979
59. cott DB, McClure J: Selective epidural analgesia (correspondence). Lancet 1: 1410–1411, 1979
60. Shook JE, Watkins WD, Camporesi EM: Differential roles of opioid receptors in respiration, respiratory disease, and opiate-induced respiratory depression. Am Rev Respir Dis 142:895–909, 1990
61. Sivarajan M, Amory DW, Lindbloom LE, Schwettmann RS: Systemic and regional blood-flow changes during spinal anesthesia in the rhesus monkey. Anesthesiology 43:78–88, 1975
62. Hackel DB, Sancetta SM, Kleinerman J: Effect of hypotension due to spinal anesthesia on coronary blood flow and myocardial metabolism in man. Circulation 13:92–97, 1956
63. Reiz S, Nath S, Rais O: Effects of thoracic epidural block and prenalterol on coronary vascular resistance and myocardial metabolism in patients with coronary artery disease. Acta Anaesthesiol Scand 24:11–16, 1980
64. DiNardo JA, Bert A, Schwartz MJ, et al: Effects of vasoactive drugs on flows through left internal mammary artery and saphenous vein grafts in man. J Thorac Cardiovasc Surg 102:730–735, 1991
65. Heusch G: α-Adrenergic mechanisms in myocardial ischemia. Circulation 81:1–13, 1990
66. Reiz S, Nath S: Cardiotoxicity of local anaesthetic agents. Br J Anaesth 58:736–746, 1986
67. Wattwil M, Sundberg A, Arvill A, Lennquist C: Circulatory changes during high thoracic epidural anaesthesia–influence of sympathetic block and of systemic effect of the local anaesthetic. Acta Anaesthesiol Scand 29:849–855, 1985
68. Blomberg S, Richsten SE: Effects of thoracic epidural anaesthesia on central heamodynamics compared to cardiac beta adrenoceptor blockade in conscious rats with acute myocardial infarction. Acta Anaesthesiol Scand 34:1–7, 1990
69. Hotvedt R, Refsum H, Platou ES: Cardiac electrophysiological and hemodynamic effects of β-adrenoceptor blockade and thoracic epidural analgesia in the dog. Anesth Analg 63:817–824, 1984
70. Vandermeulen EP, Van Aken H, Vermylen J: Anticoagulants and spinal-epidural anesthesia. Anesth Analg 79:1165–1177, 1994
71. Markham JW, Lynge HN, Stahlman GEB: The syndrome of spontaneous spinal epidural hematoma: report of three cases. J Neurosurg 26:334–342, 1967
72. Waldman SD, Feldstein GS, Waldman HJ, et al: Caudal adminis-

tration of morphine sulfate in anticoagulated and thrombocytopenic patients. Anesth Analg 66:267–268, 1987

73. Odoom JA, Sih IL: Epidural analgesia and anticoagulant therapy:
experience with one thousand cases of continuous epidurals.
Anaesthesia 38:254–259, 1983

74. Owens EL, Kasten GW, Hessel EA: Spinal subarachnoid hematoma
after lumbar puncture and heparinization: a case report, review of
the literature, and discussion of anesthetic implications. Anesth
Analg 65:1201–1207, 1986

75. Brem SS, Hafler DA, Van Uitert RL, et al: Spinal subarachnoid
hematoma: a hazard of lumbar puncture resulting in reversible
paraplegia. N Engl J Med 303:1020–1021, 1981

76. Ruff RL, Dougherty JH: Complications of lumbar puncture followed by anticoagulation. Stroke 12:879–881, 1981

77. Varkey GP, Brindle GF: Peridural anaesthesia and anticoagulant
therapy. Can Anaesth Soc J 21:106–109, 1974

78. Baron HC, LaRaja RD, Rossi G, Atkinson D: Continuous epidural
analgesia in the heparinized vascular surgical patient: a retrospective review of 912 patients. J Vasc Surg 6:144–146, 1987

79. Rao TLK, El-Etr AA: Anticoagulation following placement of
epidural and subarachnoid catheters: an evaluation of neurologic
sequelae. Anesthesiology 55:618–620, 1981

80. Ho AMH, Chung DC, Joynt GM: Neuraxial blockade and hematoma
in cardiac surgery: estimating the risk of a rare adverse event that has
not (yet) occurred. Chest 117:551–555, 2000

81. Goldstein S, Dean D, Kim SJ, et al: A survey of spinal and epidural
techniques in adult cardiac surgery. J Cardiothorac Vasc Anesth
15:158–168, 2001

82. Zenati MA, Paiste J, Williams JP, et al: Minimally invasive coronary bypass without general endotracheal anesthesia. Ann Thorac
Surg 72:1380–1382, 2001

83. Karagoz HY, Sonmez B, Bakkaloglu B, et al: Coronary artery bypass grafting in the conscious patient without endotracheal general anesthesia. Ann Thorac Surg 70:91–96, 2000

84. O'Connor CJ, Tuman KJ: Epidural anesthesia and analgesia for
coronary artery bypass graft surgery: still forbidden territory? (editorial). Anesth Analg 93:523–525, 2001

85. Riedel BJCJ: Regional anesthesia for major cardiac and noncardiac
surgery: more than just a strategy for effective analgesia? (editorial). J Cardiothorac Vasc Anesth 15:279–281, 2001

86. Castellano JM, Durbin CG: Epidural analgesia and cardiac surgery;
worth the risk? (editorial). Chest 117:305–307, 2000

John E. Ellis, M.D.
James F. McKinsey, M.D.

Regional Anesthesia for Endovascular Procedures

5

INTRODUCTION

There has been an explosion in the use of endovascular therapy for aortic and peripheral vascular disease. Approximately half of patients with abdominal aortic aneurysm (AAA) appear to be candidates for endovascular repair. Experienced centers have not noted a decrease in open AAA repair accompanying the growth of endovascular AAA repair (endoAAAR) programs (1). This growth in endovascular repair has been occasioned by hopes of lower morbidity and mortality and shorter hospital stays and convalescence. In addition, manufacturers have driven the growth of endovascular procedures. Despite the shorter length of stay (LOS) after endoAAAR, the costs of the implant (~$9000) and radiologic procedures actually may result in higher costs (~$7200 more) than open surgery (2); anesthesia costs, though, are lower for endovascular repair.

Vascular surgeons, cardiac surgeons, interventional radiologists, and/or cardiologists (with turf battles not uncommon) may perform procedures. When they are performed outside of the main operating room (ours are performed by vascular surgeons in a specialized suite built in the ambulatory operating rooms), appropriate equipment must be provided. This may include a blood refrigerator, the ability to obtain arterial blood gases and other labs, fluid warmers, forced-air warming, etc. When faced with new technologies, clinicians caring for patients undergoing such procedures must exercise good judgment. That means

Regional Anesthesia for Cardiothoracic Surgery, edited by Mark Chaney, Lippincott Williams & Wilkins, Baltimore © 2002.

being prepared for the rare disaster, especially during the "learning curves" of new practitioners.

Most recently, several series with long-term follow-up have high-lighted some limitations of endoAAAR. Concerns have arisen over the expense of repeated postoperative surveillance, because further aneurys-mal dilation and endoleaks may occur. Additionally, procedural-related mortality may not be as low as initially suggested, especially as indica-tions are expanded and the procedures are used in sicker patients (3).

EPIDEMIOLOGY AND PATHOPHYSIOLOGY OF ABDOMINAL AORTIC ANEURYSM

There are approximately 200,000 new cases of AAA diagnosed annu-ally, with approximately 45,000 patients undergoing surgical repair per year in the United States. A population-based study of 6,386 men and women in Norway in 1994–1995 used ultrasound to measure renal and infrarenal aortic diameters; an aneurysm was present in 263 (8.9%) men and 74 (2.2%) women ($p < 0.001$). Risk factors for aneurysm included advanced age, smoking for more than 40 years, the need (ever) for anti-hypertensive medication, a low serum HDL cholesterol, a high level of plasma fibrinogen, and a low blood platelet count. This study indicates that risk factors for atherosclerosis are also associated with increased risk for AAA (4).

AAA represents a dilation of the abdominal aorta generally below the level of the renal arteries. The risk of rupture of the AAA is directly related to the luminal diameter of the aortic aneurysm. The aneurysm can develop an inner lining of mural thrombus thereby decreasing the effective luminal diameter, but the size of the mural thrombus has not been shown to significantly decrease the risk of rupture. The risk of aortic rupture is related only to the absolute diameter of the aortic aneurysm sac. The risk of rupture increases once the aneurysm is greater than 4.5 to 5 cm in diameter. Generally, it has been recommended that good-risk patients with aneurysms greater than 4.5 to 5 cm should be considered for surgical repair.

Traditional surgery for ruptured AAA is still associated with mor-tality approaching 50%, roughly an order of magnitude greater than elective AAA surgery. Risk factors for mortality in patients with rup-ture include advanced age, a high APACHE (Acute Physiology and Chronic Health Evaluation) II score, low initial hematocrit, and preop-erative cardiac arrest (5). Unfortunately, in more than 70% of patients in this series from the Mayo Clinic, the diagnosis of AAA was unknown. These data reinforce the importance of screening the high-risk popula-tion to permit elective repair.

CONVENTIONAL SURGERY

Conventional surgical repair entails either a midline abdominal incision or a left flank retroperitoneal incision for exposure of the abdominal aorta. Dissection is carried out to the region of the aorta above the area of the aneurysmal dilation and then the aorta is exposed down to the distal aorta or the iliac arteries depending on the distal extent of the aneurysmal dilation. In isolated cases in which there is also concomitant iliac atherosclerotic stenotic disease, aorta-bifemoral bypass grafting has been recommended. Conventional open aneurysm repair requires cross clamping the aorta with the potential for significant increase in afterload resistance during the time of aortic cross-clamp, and then reperfusion with significant hemodynamic and metabolic changes during the time of aortic cross-clamp release (6). Intraoperative blood loss during open AAA repair varies between 500 to several thousand milliliters of blood depending on the size and complexity of the AAA.

The postoperative course many times requires admission to the intensive care unit for several days and hospital admission for 5 to 7 days. The postoperative recovery period after the open repair can be several months. The perioperative mortality for elective conventional aneurysm repair has been reported between 2% and 5% in good-risk patients, and 6.2% in elective cases in the state of California in 1990–1994 (7). If the patient presents with a ruptured AAA, the perioperative mortality can be as high as 50% to 70%. Perioperative morbidity also includes myocardial infarction, pulmonary dysfunction, renal failure, injury to the ureter, bowel ischemia or infarction, and erectile dysfunction in some men.

ENDOVASCULAR TECHNIQUES

In 1991, Juan Parodi reported a small series of high-risk patients who underwent minimally invasive endoluminal repair of their aortic aneurysm through catheter delivery of grafts from remote cut-downs in the femoral arteries (8). His initial report triggered significant interest within the vascular surgical community on the minimally invasive repair of AAA. Initially, homemade devices were used to bridge the area of the aortic aneurysm with an expandable stent and Dacron-coated grafts.

Commercially produced grafts initially started clinical trials in the United States in 1994 with the Endovascular Technologies (EVT) device, which consisted of unibody construction with hook attachment sites at both the proximal and distal aspect of the graft (9). These hooks were embedded with balloons into the aorta and iliac vessels, mimicking the effect of conventional surgical suturing. The body of the graft was unsupported, again consistent with the conventional open aortic aneurysm repair. Other graft designs quickly became available, which involved the use of supported grafts with first expandable stainless steel stents and then the Nitinol stent that implemented the use of the radial force of the stent to hold the stent graft in place. Generally, a neck below the renal arteries of approximately 15 mm is required for adequate fixation of the stent graft to the infrarenal aorta. The distal attachment of these grafts would either be to the distal abdominal aorta if an adequate neck was noted above the aortic bifurcation or in most cases into the common iliac vessels distal to the aneurysmal dilation.

The technique for implantation of the endovascular aortic grafts generally requires bilateral common femoral artery or iliac artery cutdown in the supine position. Arterial sheaths between 16 and 27 French are then advanced into the iliac arteries and up into the AAA sac. This can be performed using local anesthetic, spinal, epidural, or general endotracheal anesthetic, as discussed below. If the patient has small common femoral or external iliac arteries, the introducer sheath may be too large to safely advance to the abdominal aorta. In these cases, a retroperitoneal cut-down to the distal common iliac artery or the proximal external iliac artery can be performed to access a more suitable caliber vessel for graft implantation. This can be done with a small retroperitoneal incision and dissection down to the iliac vessels and the suturing of a synthetic conduit onto the common iliac artery or the junction of the common and external iliac artery. The graft is then introduced through this conduit and deployed either into the common iliac artery or in some cases actually into the conduit itself. The conduit can then either be ligated or implanted into the femoral artery as an ilial femoral bypass graft. In isolated cases with extension of the aneurysm to the bifurcation of the common iliac into the external and internal iliac artery, embolization of the internal iliac artery or reimplantation of the internal iliac artery into the external iliac artery by a retroperitoneal cut-down have been employed and placement of the iliac stent graft into the external iliac artery.

Preimplantation calibrated angiography is required to identify the renal vessels, the potential for an accessory renal artery, the length from the renal arteries to the aortic bifurcation, and then the distance from the aortic bifurcation to the bifurcation of the common iliac artery to the external and internal iliac artery (Figure 5–1). Dye loads average from 120 to 200 cc, depending on whether calibrated angiography is performed at the same time. These measurements coupled with the diameter measurements allow the selection of the appropriate sized endovascular stent graft. The device is then positioned just below the renal artery orifices (Figures 5–2 through 5–4) and then fully deployed (Figure 5–5). Each type of stent graft has a unique method of deployment and specialized training is required for each device.

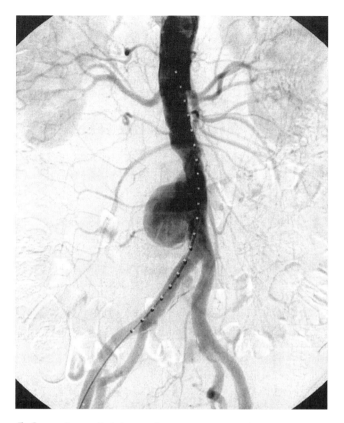

FIGURE 5–1. Infrarenal abdominal aortic aneurysm that ends above aortic bifurcation.

Major complications in endovascular stent grafting have included aneurysm rupture during the time of graft implantation, renal insufficiency secondary to contrast use, and the late complications include migration of the graft with changes in configuration of the aortic aneurysm sac, endoleak, or late AAA rupture.

Endoleak is defined as a persistent perfusion of the aneurysm sac through attachment site leakage points (Type 1 endoleak) or through lumbar or mesenteric artery branches (Type 2 endoleak). A tear in the fabric of the aortic stent graft or a modular disconnect between the pieces of the endovascular aortic stent graft is classified as a Type 3 endoleak. The significance of aortic endoleak is still uncertain. It has been shown that Type 1 endoleaks have a high potential for aortic expansion or even rupture and should be repaired with an additional stent, covered stent, or conversion to an open AAA repair. The significance of Type 2 endoleak is uncertain. The general consensus is that in the pres-

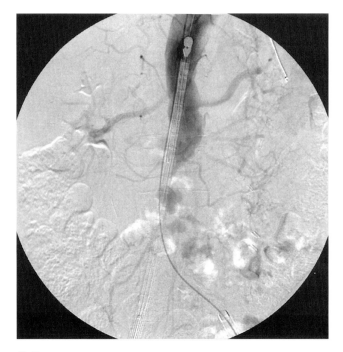

FIGURE 5–2. Positioning of aortic stent graft above the renal arteries before deployment.

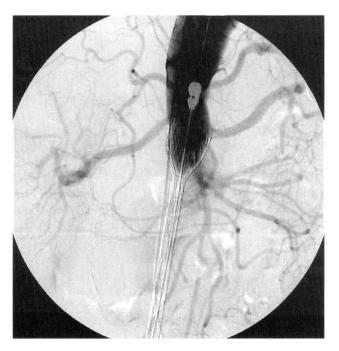

FIGURE 5–3. Initial deployment of the aortic stent graft with pulling the graft down to the perirenal position.

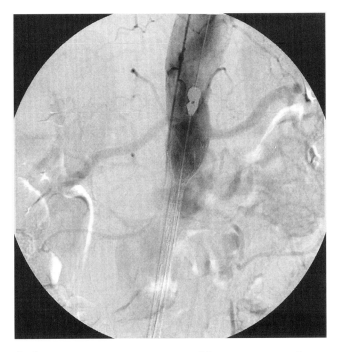

FIGURE 5–4.   Final infrarenal positioning of the aortic stent graft.

ence of a Type 2 endoleak the patient should be followed with serial CT scans and only intervened upon if there are signs of progression or enlargement of the aortic aneurysm sac. Endoleaks may require subsequent repair in a significant percentage (up to 10%) of patients (10).

The potential for the need for retroperitoneal cut-down to the iliac arteries or worst case scenario injury to the iliac vessels or the aortic aneurysm itself, necessitates that these procedures be performed in a setting that is suitable for either urgent transfer to the operating facility or preferably within the operating room itself. This way, if either open aortic conversion or iliac repair is required, this can be accomplished with greatest efficiency and safety. One of the major FDA approved devices has shown that there is approximately a 0.8 % risk of rupture in the perioperative or long-term postoperative period after aortic stent graft placement. Many of these cases are actually due to lack of follow-up and failure to intervene on changes of the aortic morphology that could have prevented AAA rupture.

Follow-up is critical in the patients undergoing endovascular aortic stent grafting. Generally, patients are followed with plain x-ray and serial CT scans at 1, 3, 6, 12, 18, and 24 months, and then yearly. This differs from the standard open aneurysm repair in which the patient may receive an ultrasound or no follow-up whatsoever except for physical ex-

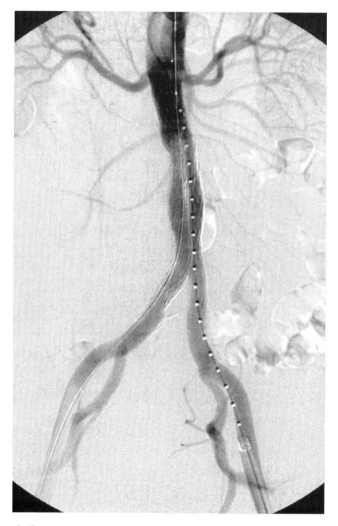

FIGURE 5–5.   Final angiogram after deployment of the aortic stent graft.

amination. The follow-up CT scans after endovascular aortic stent grafts are to detect signs of endoleak, aneurysmal sac enlargement, or graft migration. Graft migration can be caused by a technical problem with the stent graft itself or by changes in the configuration of the aortic aneurysm as it decreases in size from lack of perfusion and then kinking or migration of the graft. Many late complications of aortic stent grafting can be repaired through endovascular techniques of embolization or by adding more cuffs without necessitating open surgical conversion.

There are still many questions regarding the long-term patency and durability of endovascular aortic stent grafts (11) but the preliminary data appear good. Changes in the design and configuration of aortic stent graft have shown significant improvement in the patency and ability to implant these devices into the abdominal aorta. As the grafts continue to progress into their 3rd and 4th generation, the authors are optimistic that this will continue to improve and become a safe and effective way of managing AAA.

GOALS OF ANESTHESIA FOR ENDOVASCULAR ANEURYSM REPAIR

As in open AAA repair, the primary goal of perioperative management is to preserve organ function. This is particularly important, because endoAAAR patients may be sicker and have more end-organ disease than candidates for open repair (12).

Even when performed under monitored anesthesia care, preparation for endoAAAR must anticipate significant blood loss and fluid requirements. In a series of 47 patients (from one of the most experienced centers in the United States), the average blood loss was 623 ml (range, 100–2500 ml), and fluid requirements averaged 2491 ml (13). Therefore, the choice of a local or regional anesthetic may still require placement of invasive monitors in patients.

At the time of deployment, mild hypotension and lack of patient movement are important goals. In early series, induction of ventricular fibrillation or atrial-ventricular block with adenosine was used to induce brief asystole. These are more feasible under general anesthesia compared to regional anesthesia. However, more recently, mild hypotension is used, which can be induced with infusions of vasodilators such as nitroglycerin (14). In the patient receiving regional anesthesia or monitored anesthesia care, brief induction of general anesthesia with a bolus of propofol and mask ventilation may be indicated.

A variety of anesthetic techniques have been used for endoAAAR, including general, epidural, combined epidural/spinal (15), spinal, and continuous spinal (16). Because most endoAAAR are associated with less hemodynamic stress, endocrine stress, cytokine release, decline in respiratory function, and prolonged convalescence compared to open repair, regional anesthesia might have less incremental benefit in endoAAAR. Of course, controversy persists even for open AAA repair, as to whether or not regional anesthesia improves outcome (17).

MANAGING INTRAOPERATIVE COMPLICATIONS

EndoAAAR, while likely representing a significant advance, is not benign. In one English series of 221 patients, 30-day mortality was 11.3%

(18). Most deaths occurred in high-risk patients (63% of this group had at least one of these features: creatinine > 150 micromol/L, ischemic heart disease, poor left ventricular function, respiratory function $< 50\%$ of predicted, ruptured or symptomatic AAA, contraindication to or failed open repair, or age > 80 years).

A recent registry suggests that endovascular repair may not be so benign in the highest risk patients. The 1-year cumulative survival for patients unfit for surgery and patients unfit for general anesthesia was 20% and 23%, respectively. "The risks of endovascular aneurysm repair might, therefore, exceed that of nonoperative management. Caution should be used when advising these patients about endovascular repair (19)." In a series of 64 Dutch patients, advanced age and medical co-morbidity were associated with increased risk for perioperative complications and death. "Additional perioperative procedures are usually well tolerated. With greater experience in endovascular AAA grafting, the incidence of complications and endoleaks decreased (20)."

Rupture may rarely occur during endoAAAR. In a case report, intraoperative monitored rupture, despite rapid inflation of a proximal balloon to effectively "cross-clamp" the aorta, was associated with hemorrhagic shock typical of ruptures occurring outside the hospital. In this patient, endotracheal intubation was performed after rupture because a regional anesthetic technique was originally chosen (21). We are more likely to provide general anesthesia for patients with complicated anatomy (especially iliac arteries), where conversion might be more likely.

Misdeployment may result in immediate onset of visceral ischemia. Alternatively, atheroembolization may occur with resultant ischemic complications (22). Blood loss may be considerable in patients with severely diseased and tortuous femoral or iliac arteries. Injury to these arteries may require repair. A proactive approach in such a patient with severe iliac disease was described in a case report. In this report, an open iliac artery reconstruction (under regional anesthesia) was initially performed, followed by stent deployment via the reconstructed artery (23). Other workers have suggested arterial access via the brachial or carotid arteries.

As mentioned above, mortality in patients with ruptured AAA remains high after traditional surgery. Recently, the group from Montefiore in New York has reported significantly better results with a novel, multifaceted approach that includes endovascular repair with a proprietary device, hypotensive hemostasis, and limited fluid resuscitation (24). Using this approach, 23 of 25 patients with ruptured aortoiliac aneurysms (18 aortic, 7 iliac) survived. The authors state: "Under local anesthesia, a transbrachial guidewire was placed under fluoroscopic control in the supraceliac aorta. A 40-mm balloon catheter was inserted over this guidewire and inflated only if the blood pressure was less than

50 mm Hg, before or after the induction of anesthesia. Fluoroscopic angiography was used to determine the suitability for endovascular graft repair. When possible, a prepared, "one-size-fits-most" endovascular aortounifemoral stented PTFE graft was used, combined with occlusion of the contralateral common iliac artery and femorofemoral bypass." Balloon inflation for proximal control was required in only 9 of the 25 patients. Twenty patients were treated with endovascular grafts; 5 patients required open repair. The ruptured aneurysm was excluded in all 25 patients; 23 survived. Two deaths occurred in patients who received endovascular grafts with serious comorbidities. The surviving patients who received endovascular grafts had a median hospital stay of 6 days, and the preoperative symptoms resolved in all patients. This approach tends to contradict traditional notions of the importance of aggressive volume resuscitation and normalization of blood pressure. However, this approach has been adapted from one shown successful in surgical patients suffering penetrating trauma (25). The endovascular approach to patients with ruptured AAA may be limited because of the need for time-consuming measurement (angiography) and the expense of keeping multiple sized grafts in inventory. Future studies will define the role of endovascular therapy in emergent and rupture situations.

Traditional surgery for thoracic aortic aneurysm continues to be associated with higher morbidity and mortality than infrarenal AAA. The analysis of large databases suggests that population-based perioperative mortality is higher than that reported in series from selected institutions (26). Mortality may approach 20%; risk factors include diabetes mellitus, cerebrovascular disease, and renal insufficiency. Median hospital charges ($64,000) are also high. Therefore, endovascular thoracoabdominal aortic aneurysm repair (endoTAAR) has been advocated as an alternative to open surgery with its stresses and frequent complications. Complications may be lower with endovascular approaches. The recent UCLA experience in 26 patients resulted in 25 successful thoracic aortic stent deployments, no conversion to open surgery, and only one peri-procedural death at 30 days, though after an average follow-up of 9 months, nearly one-quarter were dead (27). Additionally, blood loss averaged only 450 cc, ICU stay 1 day, and hospital stay 5 days in the uncomplicated cases (22 of 26). One case of paraplegia occurred, consistent with other series suggesting that while paraplegia still may occur after endoTAAR, its incidence seems reduced compared to open TAAR (28). One approach to attempt to lessen paraplegia after endoTAAR has been to place a temporary stent under somatosensory-evoked potential (SSEP) monitoring; if SSEP is unchanged, then the thinking goes, a permanent stent may be placed (29). In this study, none of 16 patients had SSEP changes with stent deployment. However, motor-evoked potential monitoring would seem more appropriate for monitoring function of the anterior spinal column (30). Drainage of cerebrospinal fluid (CSF) may be performed in attempt to rescue patients with paraplegia, as has been reported after open TAAR. Several authors have reported successful treatment of paraplegia following endoTAAR (31). The use of a single continuous subarachnoid catheter, first for local anesthetic injection and later for prophylactic removal of CSF, has been described during endoTAAR (32). Aspiration of CSF does not result in loss of the sensory or motor blockade if performed 15 to 20 minutes after local anesthetic instillation. Paraplegia has also been reported after endoAAAR; atheroembolization to the spinal cord appears to have been the underlying cause (33).

COMPLICATIONS OF ANESTHESIA

EndoAAAR is often advocated for patients with chronic obstructive pulmonary disease. Respiratory function is better preserved after endoAAAR under general anesthesia compared to openAAA repair under general anesthesia (34). While regional anesthesia may offer pulmonary benefits for patients undergoing open repair, it is not so clearly the case in endoAAAR. This may be because the hemodynamic (35) and endocrine metabolic response to endoAAAR is far less than for open repair. "The open group had a 9.6-fold increase in epinephrine release, which was significantly higher than the 1.6-fold increase in the endovascular group ($p < 0.05$). Elevations in cortisol were also significantly higher in the open group. Early postoperative nutritional derangements, as reflected by the levels of retinol-binding protein, were far less in the endovascular group than in the open group (36)." Therefore, the potential amount of stress reduction produced by using regional anesthesia for endoAAAR is likely to be much less than for open AAAR.

Local sedation techniques have been used successfully for endoAAAR (37) as well as endoTAAR (38). Indeed, it has been suggested that the use of epidural anesthesia, as opposed to local sedation, may prolong stay and costs after ambulatory endovascular repair, perhaps because of greater administration of intravenous fluids in the epidural group (39). However, interpretation of this and other retrospective studies may be confounded by the likely selection of epidural techniques for more extensive, complicated procedures, and those earlier in the "learning curve." Similarly, the validity of retrospective studies of outcome after endoAAAR under general anesthesia versus regional anesthesia techniques may be limited. One German retrospective study suggests that "the use of pulmonary artery pressure monitoring, incidence of intraoperative hypotensive episodes, and postoperative intensive care was more frequent with general anesthesia" for endoAAAR. The authors do emphasize, however, that "regional and local anesthesia with sedation are feasible alternatives to general endotracheal anesthesia for minimally invasive treatment of aortic aneurysms by endovascular stenting. However, invasive monitoring and close postoperative monitoring are strongly recommended with either method (40)."

In traditional femoral-distal surgery, failure rates as high as 10% for spinal and 15% for epidural anesthesia have been reported (41). Failure was defined as the need to convert to general anesthesia. In our experience, most conversions from regional to general have occurred either during long procedures when patients became restless, or because of complications of the procedure (i.e., hemorrhage), which required aggressive management.

Anticoagulation management can complicate regional anesthesia in endoAAAR patients. One disadvantage of using epidural or continuous spinal catheter techniques is the need to wait until heparin effect has dissipated before removing the catheter. In most patients, postoperative pain is not a significant issue after successful endoAAAR, particularly if the groin incisions have been infiltrated with local anesthetic. Therefore, maintaining an epidural or subarachnoid catheter after surgery is not generally necessary to provide analgesia, unless more extensive adjuvant procedures, such as iliac artery repair, have been performed. Obviously, the normal cautions that apply to regional anesthesia in patients receiving preoperative anticoagulation or antiplatelet therapy apply to those undergoing endoAAAR (42).

SUMMARY

Endovascular repair likely represents an advance in care, but not a panacea. Clinicians caring for these patients must be prepared for complications. Regional and local anesthesia with sedation may be a key part of the management of these patients if the caveats discussed above are kept in mind. As the grafts continue to progress into their 3rd and 4th generation, the authors are optimistic that this will continue to improve and become a routine, safe, and effective way of managing abdominal aortic aneurysms.

References

1. Wolf YG, et al: Endovascular repair of abdominal aortic aneurysms: Eligibility rate and impact on the rate of open repair. J Vasc Surg 32(3):519–523, 2000

2. Clair DG, et al: An evaluation of the costs to health care institutions of endovascular aortic aneurysm repair. J Vasc Surg 32(1):148–152, 2000

3. Bush RL et al: Mid-term results after endovascular repair of the abdominal aortic aneurysm. J Vasc Surg 33:S70–76, 2001

4. Singh K, Bonaa KH, Jacobsen BK, Bjork L, Solberg S: Prevalence of and risk factors for abdominal aortic aneurysms in a population-based study: The Tromso Study. Am J Epidemiol 154(3):236–244, 2001

5. Noel AA, Gloviczki P, Cherry KJ Jr, Bower TC, Panneton JM, Mozes GI, Harmsen WS, Jenkins GD, Hallett JW Jr: Ruptured abdominal aortic aneurysms: The excessive mortality rate of conventional repair. J Vasc Surg 34(1):41–46, 2001

6. Gelman S: The pathophysiology of aortic cross-clamping and unclamping. Anesthesiology 82(4):1026–1060, 1995

7. Manheim LM, Sohn MW, Feinglass J, Ujiki M, Parker MA, Pearce WH: Hospital vascular surgery volume and procedure mortality rates in California, 1982–1994. J Vasc Surg 28(1):45–56, 1998

8. Parodi JC, Palmaz JC, Barone HD: Transfemoral intraluminal graft implantation for abdominal aortic aneurysms. Ann Vasc Surg 5(6):491–499, 1991

9. Moore WS, Vescera CL: Repair of abdominal aortic aneurysm by transfemoral endovascular graft placement. Ann Surg 220(3):331–339, 1994

10. May J, et al: Life-table analysis of primary and assisted success following endoluminal repair of abdominal aortic aneurysms: The role of supplementary endovascular intervention in improving outcome. Eur J Vasc Endovasc Surg 19(6):648–655, 2000

11. Ohki T, Veith FJ, Shaw P, Lipsitz E, Suggs WD, Wain RA, Bade M, Mehta M, Cayne N, Cynamon J, Valldares J, McKay J: Increasing incidence of midterm and long-term complications after endovascular graft repair of abdominal aortic aneurysms: a note of caution based on a 9-year experience. Ann Surg 234(3):323–335, 2001

12. Nishimura M, et al: Endovascular stent graft placement for patients with aortic aneurysm and end-organ dysfunction. ASAIO J 44(5):M511–515, 1998

13. Henretta JP, et al: Feasibility of endovascular repair of abdominal aortic aneurysms with local anesthesia with intravenous sedation. J Vasc Surg 29(5):793–798, 1999

14. Bernard EO, et al: Nitroglycerin to control blood pressure during endovascular stent-grafting of descending thoracic aortic aneurysms. J Vasc Surg 31(4):790–793, 2000

15. Aadahl P, et al: Regional anesthesia for endovascular treatment of abdominal aortic aneurysms. J Endovasc Surg 4(1):56–61, 1997

16. Mathes DD, Kern JA: Continuous spinal anesthetic technique for endovascular aortic stent graft surgery. J Clin Anesth 12(6):487–490, 2000

17. Baron JF, Bertrand M, Barre E, Godet G, Mundler O, Coriat P, Viars P: Combined epidural and general anesthesia versus general anesthesia for abdominal aortic surgery. Anesthesiology 75(4):611–618, 1991

18. Walker SR, et al: Mortality rates following endovascular repair of abdominal aortic aneurysms. J Endovasc Surg 6(3):233–238, 1999

19. Laheij RJ, van Marrewijk CJ: Endovascular stenting of abdominal aortic aneurysm in patients unfit for elective open surgery. Lancet 356(9232):832, 2000

20. Cuypers P, et al: Complications in the endovascular repair of abdominal aortic aneurysms: A risk factor analysis. Eur J Vasc Endovasc Surg 18(3):245–252, 1999

21. Moskowitz DM, et al: Intraoperative rupture of an abdominal aortic aneurysm during an endovascular stent-graft procedure. Can J Anaesth 46(9):887–890, 1999

22. Lindholt JS, et al: Fatal late multiple emboli after endovascular treatment of abdominal aortic aneurysm. Case report. Int Angiol 17(4):241–243, 1998

23. Chuter TA, Reilly LM: Surgical reconstruction of the iliac arteries prior to endovascular aortic aneurysm repair. J Endovasc Surg 4(3):307–311, 1997

24. Ohki T, Veith FJ: Endovascular grafts and other image-guided catheter-based adjuncts to improve the treatment of ruptured aortoiliac aneurysms. Ann Surg 232(4):466–479, 2000

25. Siegel JH, Veech RL, Lessard MR., Brochu JG, Brisson J, Carli PA, de la Coussaye JE, Riou B, Bickell WH, Pepe PE, Mattox K: L. Immediate versus delayed fluid resuscitation in patients with trauma. N Engl J Med 332:681–683, 1995

26. Derrow AE, Seeger JM, Dame DA, Carter RL, Ozaki CK, Flynn TC, Huber TS: The outcome in the United States after thoracoabdominal aortic aneurysm repair, renal artery bypass, and mesenteric revascularization. J Vasc Surg 34(1):54–61, 2001

27. White RA, Donayre CE, Walot I, Lippmann M, Woody J, Lee J, Kim N, Kopchok GE, Fogarty TJ: Endovascular exclusion of descending thoracic aortic aneurysms and chronic dissections: Initial clinical results with the AneuRx device. J Vasc Surg 33(5):927–934, 2001

28. Ehrlich M, et al: Endovascular stent graft repair for aneurysms on the descending thoracic aorta. Ann Thorac Surg 66(1):19–24; discussion 24–25, 1998

29. Ishimaru S, et al: Preliminary report on prediction of spinal cord ischemia in endovascular stent graft repair of thoracic aortic

aneurysm by retrievable stent graft. J Thorac Cardiovasc Surg 115(4):811–818, 1998

30. Meylaerts SA, Jacobs MJ, van Iterson V, De Haan P, Kalkman CJ: Comparison of transcranial motor evoked potentials and somatosensory evoked potentials during thoracoabdominal aortic aneurysm repair. Ann Surg 230(6):742–749, 1999

31. Tiesenhausen K, et al: Cerebrospinal fluid drainage to reverse paraplegia after endovascular thoracicaortic aneurysm repair. J Endovasc Ther 7(2):132–135, 2000

32. Kim SS, Leibowitz AB: Endovascular thoracic aortic aneurysm repair using a single catheter for spinal anesthesia and cerebrospinal fluid drainage. J Cardio Vasc Anesth 15(1):88–89, 2001

33. Rockman CB, Riles TS, Landis R: Lower extremity paraparesis or paraplegia subsequent to endovascular management of abdominal aortic aneurysms. J Vasc Surg 33(1):178–180, 2001

34. Boyle JR, e al: Improved respiratory function and analgesia control after endovascular AAA repair. J Endovasc Surg 4(1):62–65, 1997

35. Kahn RA, et al: Endovascular aortic repair is associated with greater hemodynamic stability compared with open aortic reconstruction. J Cardiothorac Vasc Anesth 13(1):42–46, 1999

36. Salartash K, et al: Comparison of open transabdominal AAA repair with endovascular AAA repair in reduction of postoperative stress response. Ann Vasc Surg 15(1):53–59, 2001

37. Papazoglou K, et al: Endovascular abdominal aortic aneurysm repair with percutaneous transfemoral prostheses deployment under local anaesthesia. Initial experience with a new, simple-to-use tubular and bifurcated device in the first 27 cases. Eur J Vasc Endovasc Surg 17(3):202–207, 1999

38. Lachat M, Pfammatter T, Turina M: Transfemoral endografting of thoracic aortic aneurysm under local anesthesia: A simple, safe and fast track procedure. Vasa 28(3):204–206, 1999

39. Shindelman LE, et al: Ambulatory endovascular surgery: Cost advantage and factors influencing its safe performance. J Endovasc Surg 6(2):160–167, 1999.

40. Eberle B, et al: Anesthesia in endovascular treatment of aortic aneurysm. Results and perioperative risks. Anaesthesist 45(10): 931–940, 1996

41. Bode RH Jr, Lewis KP, Zarich SW, Pierce ET, Roberts M, Kowalchuk GJ, Satwicz PR, Gibbons GW, Hunter JA, Espanola CC: Cardiac outcome after peripheral vascular surgery. Comparison of general and regional anesthesia. Anesthesiology 84(1):3–13, 1996

42. Tzeng GF: Hemostatic intervention and regional anesthesia for vascular surgery. Prob Anesthesia 11(2):207–223, 1999

Gregory B. Hammer, M.D.

6 | Regional Anesthesia for Pediatric Cardiac Surgery

INTRODUCTION

The use of regional anesthesia in combination with general anesthesia for children undergoing cardiac surgery is the subject of a growing number of publications and presentations. Reported benefits of regional anesthesia in patients having cardiac surgery include attenuation of the neuroendocrine response to surgical stress, improved postoperative pulmonary function, enhanced cardiovascular stability, and improved postoperative analgesia. To the extent that regional anesthesia facilitates early tracheal extubation in cardiac surgical patients, complications and costs associated with postoperative mechanical ventilation may be reduced. These benefits must, however, be weighed against the adverse effects that may accompany the use of regional anesthesia. These include hypotension, postoperative respiratory depression, and epidural hematoma formation. In this article, the benefits and risks of regional anesthesia in infants and children having open heart surgery are reviewed. In addition, specific techniques currently in use are described.

THE BENEFITS OF REGIONAL ANESTHESIA IN CARDIAC SURGERY

Adverse physiologic responses that occur during and after cardiac surgery include alterations in circulatory (tachycardia, hypertension, vasoconstriction), metabolic (increased catabolism), immunologic (impaired immune response), and hemostatic (platelet activation) systems (1, 2). Together, these changes are referred to as the "stress response."

Regional Anesthesia for Cardiothoracic Surgery, edited by Mark Chaney, Lippincott Williams & Wilkins, Baltimore © 2002.

The stress response associated with cardiac surgery in neonates may be profound and is associated with increased morbidity and mortality. Anand et al. measured the stress response during and after cardiac surgery in 15 neonates anesthetized with halothane and morphine (3). They found elevated plasma concentrations of epinephrine, norepinephrine, cortisol, glucagon, and beta endorphin in all patients, accompanied by hyperglycemia and lactic acidemia. The 4 deaths in the study group occured in neonates with the greatest stress responses.

Bromage et al. first demonstrated in 1971 that the stress response associated with major abdominal and thoracic surgery could be attenuated with epidural blockade (4). Since then, several investigators have shown that the use of regional anesthesia during and after cardiac surgery (i.e., intraoperative anesthesia and postoperative analgesia) may decrease the stress response as well as morbidity and mortality (5–12). Regional anesthesia (intrathecal or epidural blockade) with opioids and/or local anesthetics appears to be more effective in inhibiting the stress response associated with surgery than intravenous (IV) opioids. For example, epidural fentanyl is more effective than IV fentanyl in reducing the stress response after thoracotomy in adults (13). Epidural morphine administration was shown to attenuate the adverse decrease in T3 (liothyronine) concentration in children undergoing open heart surgery compared with general anesthesia alone (10). Epidural anesthesia with bupivacaine suppresses the increase in serum catecholamines, glucose, and adrenocorticotropic hormone (ACTH) more effectively than intravenous fentanyl in infants (11). Epidural local anesthetics may be more efficacious than opioids in attenuating the stress response (12). In a study of fetal lambs, total spinal anesthesia completely blocked the stress response to surgical manipulation and cardiopulmonary bypass (14).

Gruber et al. studied the effects on the stress response of intravenous fentanyl and midazolam on 45 infants undergoing cardiac surgery (15). Patients were randomized to receive fentanyl 0.05–0.10 mg/kg with or without midazolam 0.10 mg/kg/hr during the surgery. Plasma epinephrine, norepinephrine, cortisol, adrenocortical hormone, glucose, and lactate were measured at five intervals during and after surgery. In all groups, plasma epinephrine, norepinephrine, cortisol, glucose, and lactate concentrations were significantly greater at the completion of surgery than prior to skin incision. The authors concluded that fentanyl dosing strategies, with or without midazolam, do not prevent a hormonal or metabolic stress response in infants undergoing cardiac surgery.

Additional benefits that may be attributed to regional anesthesia include improved pulmonary function, greater circulatory stability, and reduced pain scores. Several randomized, controlled studies in adults have shown that patients receiving epidural analgesia have better pulmonary function after thoracic surgery than those treated with intravenous opioids. Thoracic epidural opioids are associated with improved pulmonary function following chest surgery compared with IV opioids (16). In a study comparing thoracic epidural meperidine to IV meperidine for postoperative analgesia, the patients receiving epidural infusions had significantly greater forced expiratory volume (FEV) and forced vital capacity (FVC), and were more cooperative with deep breathing maneuvers than those in the IV meperidine group (17). Thoracic epidural anesthesia may also improve respiratory performance postoperatively by effecting an improvement in diaphragmatic function (18).

Several studies in infants and children demonstrate reduced opioid requirements and improved analgesia following cardiac surgery with neuraxial anesthesia. Jones et al. reported the use of intrathecal morphine for postoperative analgesia in 56 children undergoing cardiac surgery (19). Following induction of anesthesia, patients received intrathecal morphine 0.02 or 0.03 mg/kg. Tracheal extubation was performed in all patients after admission to the intensive care unit postoperatively. The duration of analgesia in both groups was similar, with two-thirds of patients requiring no supplemental analgesia for more than 18 hours.

In a retrospective review of pain control in 91 children undergoing cardiac surgery, Shayevitz et al. compared lumbar epidural morphine infusions to intravenous opioid analgesia (20). In the epidural analgesia group, lumbar epidural catheters were placed following induction of anesthesia. Preservative-free morphine sulfate was administered in a bolus dose of 0.05 mg/kg followed by a continuous infusion of 0.003 to 0.004 mg/kg/hr during and after surgery. Children in the IV analgesia group received an initial IV dose of fentanyl 0.05 mg/kg followed by a continuous infusion of 0.018 mg/kg/hr during surgery. The fentanyl infusion was reduced to 0.006 mg/kg/hr postoperatively. Patients in the epidural analgesia group had significantly lower pain scores and received significantly less supplemental analgesia postoperatively than patients in the intravenous analgesia group.

In a prospective, randomized, controlled study Rosen and Rosen evaluated the efficacy of caudal epidural morphine compared with intravenous morphine in 32 children following open cardiac surgery (21). Patients in the study group received a caudal injection of preservative-free morphine sulfate 0.075 mg/kg in the operating room following surgery but prior to awakening and tracheal extubation. Patients in the control group received IV morphine alone for post-operative analgesia. Supplemental doses of IV morphine were given to children in both groups as needed, prior to which pain scores were recorded. Children having received caudal morphine required significantly less IV morphine and had significantly lower pain scores post-operatively than patients in the control group. The mean duration of complete analgesia in children receiving caudal morphine was 6 hours (range 2–12 hours), but decreased analgesic requirements were noted for the entire 24-hour study period.

Beside having improved lung function and pain control, patients receiving epidural anesthesia have fewer opioid related side effects than patients treated with IV opioids. Patients receiving epidural anesthesia have more rapid return of bowel function following surgery compared with those receiving IV analgesics. In a recent review of 16 studies comparing epidural and systemic analgesia with regard to postoperative recovery of gastrointestinal function, all 8 studies with epidural catheter placement above T12 showed more rapid recovery of bowel function when epidural analgesia was used (22). The use of postoperative thoracic epidural analgesia with bupivacaine and morphine is associated with earlier return of gastrointestinal function and decreased hospital costs due to shortened hospital stay compared with IV morphine patient-controlled analgesia (23). A study comparing epidural versus IV fentanyl analgesia following thoracotomy also reported a lower incidence of nausea, shorter duration of ileus, and earlier hospital discharge in the epidural analgesia group (16).

ADVERSE EFFECTS OF REGIONAL ANESTHESIA FOR CARDIAC SURGERY

The most serious complications that may be associated with regional anesthesia for cardiac surgery are hypotension, respiratory depression, and epidural hematoma formation.

Systemic arterial hypotension is an undesired effect of intrathecal and epidural local anesthetic blockade. In adults with coronary artery stenosis and myocardial ischemia, local anesthetic-induced blockade of cardiac sympathetic nerve activation alleviates angina and improves coronary blood flow and ventricular function (12, 24–26). However, local anesthetic blockade to upper thoracic dermatomes produces hypotension accompanied by a decrease in coronary artery perfusion (5, 27). In infants and young children, local anesthetic blockade to T3–T5 does not produce significant changes in blood pressure nor heart rate (28). This may be attributable to decreased sympathetic innervation of the lower extremities and/or immaturity of the sympathetic nervous system in young children. In two recent studies of high spinal blockade in children undergoing open heart surgery, hemodynamic stability was demonstrated in all patients (29, 30).

Dose-dependent respiratory depression may be seen in children following the administration of epidural opioids in doses exceeding 0.05 mg/kg (31). In a study of children undergoing cardiac surgery and receiving epidural morphine in an initial dose of 0.05 mg/kg followed by a continuous infusion, however, respiratory depression did not occur (20). Several other studies in children have shown excellent analgesia and no evidence of respiratory depression when the dose of epidural morphine does not exceed 0.05 mg/kg (32–34).

Similarly, doses of intrathecal morphine of 0.02 or 0.03 mg/kg may result in significant respiratory depression following cardiac surgery in children (19). Intrathecal morphine, 0.01 mg/kg, has also been associated with respiratory depression postoperatively when combined with IV fentanyl, 0.02 mg/kg, and midazolam in adult patients undergoing cardiac surgery (35). However, in a review of children given intrathecal morphine in a dose of 0.02 mg/kg in whom no IV opioids were administered during surgery, no patient had postoperative respiratory depression (36). In addition, no child required supplemental opioid analgesia for at least 15 hours following surgery. In a recent study comparing intrathecal morphine in doses of 0.005, 0.007, and 0.010 mg/kg in children having open heart surgery, the trachea of each patient was extubated at the conclusion of surgery and no patient had signs of respiratory depression (37).

Epidural hematoma formation following epidural or spinal anesthesia is a rare but potentially catastrophic complication of neuraxial blockade in patients receiving anticoagulant therapy. In an analysis of 20 series, including more than 850,000 cases of epidural blockade and 650,000 cases of spinal anesthesia in adult patients, only 3 case reports of epidural hematoma were documented (38). Based on these data, the author estimated the risk of epidural hematoma following epidural anesthesia to be 1:150,000, and 1:220,000 following spinal anesthesia. Unfortunately, it is unknown what the incidence of clotting disorders, use of anticoagulants, or traumatic procedures was in these reports.

In a thorough review of the literature from 1906 through 1994, Vandermeulen et al. found 61 published cases of epidural or subdural hematoma following epidural or spinal anesthesia in adult patients (39). Of these 61 cases, 42 occurred in patients with impaired coagulation prior to epidural or spinal needle placement, including 25 patients receiving heparin. In 15 patients, the procedure was reported to be difficult and/or traumatic. A clotting disorder or difficult/traumatic needle placement was present in 53 of the 61 cases (87%).

In a series of over 4,000 epidural or spinal anesthetics performed prior to anticoagulation with heparin for vascular surgery, no cases of epidural hematoma were reported (40). The authors highlighted important precautions that were undertaken in these patients, including delaying surgery for 24 hours in the event of traumatic needle placement and allowing at least 60 minutes between needle placement and heparin administration. Other recommended precautions include use of the smallest dose of heparin necessary to achieve therapeutic objectives and removal of epidural catheters only when normal coagulation function has been restored (41). Epidural hematoma formation has not been reported in a patient following spinal or epidural anesthesia performed prior to cardiopulmonary bypass.

REGIONAL ANESTHESIA TECHNIQUES

A variety of techniques of neuraxial blockade have been reported in children undergoing cardiac surgery. These include intrathecal and epidural techniques utilizing opioids and/or local anesthetics. Epidural approaches include single dose ("single shot") caudals as well as thoracic, lumbar, and caudal catheter techniques.

Intrathecal (Spinal) Techniques

The use of spinal opioid analgesia as an adjunct to general anesthesia was first described by Mathews and Abrams in 1980 (42). In this report, 40 adults received intrathecal morphine in a dose of 1.5 to 4.0 mg prior to surgery. All patients remained comfortable for more than 24 hours. Subsequently, many studies have demonstrated the efficacy of spinal opioids, primarily morphine, in producing analgesia following cardiac surgery in adult patients. These reports have been summarized elsewhere (41) and are reviewed in Chapter 3 of this book. Although intrathecal morphine alone has not been shown to attenuate the stress response associated with cardiac surgery per se, it may attenuate the stress response in the immediate postoperative period (43).

In order to augment the effects of intrathecal opioids in reducing the stress response and circulatory instability in patients undergoing cardiac surgery, local anesthetics have been used in combination with intrathecal opioids. In adults, however, intrathecal injection of local anesthetics in doses needed to attain high spinal blockade results in hypotension (44). Young children, on the other hand, do not develop hypotension following high spinal blockade. Finkel et al. studied the hemodynamic effects of spinal anesthesia in children undergoing cardiac surgery (29). In this study, 30 children between the ages of 7 months and 13 years received intrathecal morphine mixed with tetracaine following induction of general anesthesia and tracheal intubation. The dose of tetracaine was adjusted for age, according to the estimated volume of cerebrospinal fluid. Patients aged 6 to 12 months received intrathecal tetracaine 2.0 mg/kg, those between the ages of 1 and 3 years received 1.0 mg/kg, and those over the age of 4 years received 0.5 mg/kg. Tetracaine was mixed with 10% dextrose to yield a 0.5% hyperbaric solution, and all patients received preservative-free morphine in a dose of 0.005 to 0.010 mg/kg. Patients were placed in a 30° head-down (Trendelenburg) position for a minimum of 10 minutes following administration of the intrathecal solution. Although there was mild slowing of the heart rate in children over age 4 years, there was no clinically significant bradycardia nor hypotension observed. Hammer et al. have also reported hemodynamic stability following intrathecal tetracaine/morphine in children undergoing cardiac surgery (30).

We currently utilize spinal anesthesia in combination with general anesthesia in children for whom tracheal extubation is planned prior to leaving the operating room following open heart surgery. Surgical procedures include, for example, repair of atrial and/or ventricular septal defects, anomalous pulmonary venous return, aortic or pulmonary valvuloplasty, right ventrical-to-pulmonary artery conduit placement or exchange, bidirectional cavopulmonary shunt, and the modified Fontan procedure. Spinal anesthetic blocks (SAB) are performed immediately after tracheal intubation (i.e., prior to placement of arterial and central venous catheters) in order to maximize the time interval between spinal needle placement and heparinization for cardiopulmonary bypass. Patients are placed with the head of the table 30° down for a minimum of 15 minutes following injection. No IV opioids are administered intraoperatively. Our dosing regimen for SAB is based on the above-referenced studies and is shown in Table 6–1.

Epidural Techniques

The use of postoperative epidural analgesia in patients undergoing open heart surgery was first described by Hoar et al. in 1976 (45). Subsequently, El-Baz and Goldin reported the use of epidural blockade initiated prior to surgical incision (9). In 1989, Rosen and Rosen first reported the efficacy of epidural morphine analgesia in children undergoing cardiac surgery (21). Since then, many studies have reported favorable results with epidural anesthesia and analgesia for cardiac surgery (41).

In general, epidural anesthesia is used in patients undergoing open heart surgery for whom tracheal extubation is planned in the operating room following the completion of surgery or shortly thereafter. The epidural technique most commonly used in children appears to be the administration of a single dose of morphine injected into the caudal epidural space. Morphine is favored for caudal epidural administration due its low lipid solubility and commensurate tendency to spread rostrally to thoracic dermatomes (46, 47). Following induction of general anesthesia and tracheal intubation, preservative-free morphine sulfate is injected in a dose of 0.05 to 0.10 mg/kg into the caudal epidural space via an epidural needle or intravenous catheter. Intravenous opioids, if administered intraoperatively, are given in restricted doses (e.g., fentanyl 0.01–0.02 mg/kg).

TABLE 6–1. Dosing regimens for spinal anesthesia

Age (years)	Tetracaine (mg/kg)	Morphine (μg/kg)
< 1	2.0	7
1–3	1.0	7
4–8	0.5	7
>8	0	10

Source: Hammer GB, Ngo K, Macario A: A retrospective examination of regional plus general anesthesia in children undergoing open heart surgery. Anesth Analg 90:1020–1024, 2000.

Alternatively, a caudal epidural catheter may be inserted to facilitate continuous administration of morphine during and after surgery. Following an initial dose of epidural morphine 0.04 mg/kg, a continuous infusion is begun in a dose of 0.0075 mg/kg/hr. The infusion is continued throughout the intraoperative period and maintained postoperatively for 48 to 72 hours. If the patient appears overly somnolent the infusion is decreased in increments of 0.0025 mg/kg/hr.[1]

In order to attenuate the stress response associated with cardiac surgery and cardiopulmonary bypass as well as optimize postoperative analgesia, a combination of epidural opioids and local anesthetic agents may be used. Although local anesthetic agents may spread to thoracic dermatomes when administered via the caudal epidural space, potentially toxic doses of local anesthetics may be required to achieve thoracic analgesia (48, 49). Thoracic epidural blockade may be achieved with greater safety and efficacy by placing the epidural catheter tip in proximity to the spinal segment associated with surgical incision. Segmental anesthesia may then be achieved with lower doses of local anesthetic than those needed when the catheter tip is distant from the surgical site. In infants, a catheter can reliably be advanced from the caudal to the thoracic epidural space (50). For example, with the infant in the lateral decubitus position, a 20-gauge epidural catheter may be inserted via an epidural needle or an 18-gauge intravenous catheter placed through the sacrococcygeal membrane and advanced 16 to 18 cm to the mid-thoracic epidural space. Minor resistance to passage of the catheter may be overcome by simple flexion or extension of the spine. If continued resistance is encountered, no attempt should be made to advance the catheter further, as the catheter may become coiled within or exit the epidural space. In older children, a thoracic epidural catheter may be inserted directly between T4 and T8 to provide intraoperative anesthesia and postoperative analgesia. As with SAB, epidural catheter placement should be performed immediately following tracheal intubation in order to maximize the time elapsed prior to heparin administration for cardiopulmonary bypass. In our practice, an initial dose of hydromorphone 0.007 to 0.008 mg/kg and 0.25% bupivacaine 0.5 ml/kg is administered. Subsequent doses of 0.25% bupivacaine 0.3 ml/kg are administered intraoperatively at approximately 90 minute intervals. No IV opioids are given during surgery. Postoperatively, a continuous infusion of 0.10% bupivacaine and hydromorphone 0.003 mg/ml is administered at a rate of 0.3 ml/kg/hr. An advantage of epidural catheter compared with "single shot" techniques is that adjustments can be made in dosing postoperatively according to the patient's level of comfort. For example, a "bolus" of epidural anesthetic agents may be given and the infusion rate increased if the patient is experiencing pain. Alternatively, the infusion

---

[1]D. Rosen—personal communication.

may be decreased if the patient becomes somnolent. Our dosing regimen for thoracic epidural anesthesia and analgesia is shown in Table 6–2.

Treatment of Side Effects

Side effects related to neuraxial opioids include nausea and vomiting, pruritus, somnolence, respiratory depression, and urinary retention. Nausea and vomiting as well as pruritus appear to be relatively uncommon in infants and are primarily seen in children over the age of 3 years. These side effects are more common with morphine compared with hydromorphone and fentanyl (51). Due to greater rostral spread, respiratory depression is also more common when morphine is used compared with hydromorphone (47, 52). Urinary retention is seen most commonly during the initial 24 hours of therapy, during which time the majority of patients have urinary catheters in place. Suggested treatment for side effects related to spinal and epidural opioids is shown in Table 6–3.

CONCLUSION

The use of epidural and spinal anesthesia in infants and children may attenuate the stress response and thereby decrease morbidity and mortality associated with cardiac surgery. In addition, the use of these regional anesthesia techniques during and after cardiac surgery may result in improved pulmonary function, greater circulatory stability, and better postoperative pain control compared with general anesthesia and postoperative intravenous opioid analgesia. To the extent that regional anesthesia may facilitate tracheal extubation in the operating room immediately following surgery, complications and the expense associated with mechanical ventilation in the postoperative period may be avoided. In those patients who undergo tracheal extubation in the intensive care unit, cost savings may be achieved due to reductions in time of mechanical ventilation and length of stay, as well as earlier resumption of a regular diet.

TABLE 6–2.　Dosing regimens for epidural anesthesia

Intraoperative dosage		Postoperative infusion
Bupivacaine 0.25%	Hydromorphone (mg/kg)	
0.5 ml/kg initially, then 0.3 ml/kg q 90 min	.007–.008	Bupivacaine 0.1% + Hydromorphone .003 mg/ml @0.3 ml/kg/hr

Source: Hammer GB, Ngo K, Macario A: A retrospective examination of regional plus general anesthesia in children undergoing open heart surgery. Anesth Analg 90:1020–1024, 2000.

The risks of epidural and spinal anesthesia in these patients include undesired side effects (nausea and vomiting, pruritus), hypotension, respiratory depression, and epidural hematoma formation. The incidence of side effects does not appear to exceed that associated with intravenous opioid analgesia. Hypotension, associated with local anesthetic spinal and epidural blockade in adult patients, is uncommon in infants and

TABLE 6–3. Treatment for side effects of neuraxial opioid administration

Side effect	Treatment	Comments
Nausea/ vomiting	Metoclopromide 0.1–0.2 mg/kg/dose IV Q 6 hours Maximum dose: 10 mg	Extrapyramidal reactions may occur but are uncommon
	Droperidol 0.025–0.05 mg/kg IV Q 6 hours prn Maximum dose: 1.25 mg	Very sedating—avoid if somnolent
	Diphenhydramine 0.5–1.0 mg/kg IV Q 6 hours prn Maximum dose: 50 mg	Very sedating—avoid if somnolent
	Ondansetron 0.1–0.2 mg/kg IV Q 6 hours prn Maximum dose: 4 mg	May substitute other 5-HT3 antagonist, e.g., granisetron or dolasetron
	Nalbuphine 0.1 mg/kg IV Q 6 hours prn	
	Naloxone 0.001–0.005 mg/kg/hr infusion	Excessive doses may compromise analgesia
	Propofol 0.001–0.010 mg/kg/min infusion	
Pruritus	Diphenhydramine 0.5–1.0 mg/kg IV Q 6 hours prn Maximum dose: 50 mg	Very sedating—avoid if somnolent
	Nalbuphine 0.1 mg/kg IV Q 6 hours prn	
	Naloxone 0.001–0.005 mg/kg/hr infusion	Excessive doses may compromise analgesia
Somnolence	Decrease epidural opioid infusion Consider low-dose naloxone infusion (above)	
Respiratory depression	Severe: Administer 100% O_2 via facemask Initiate positive pressure ventilation prn Naloxone 0.001–0.010 mg/kg IV Stop epidural infusion Subsequently/Mild-moderate depression: Increase FIO_2 Reduce epidural opioid infusion Naloxone 0.001–0.005 mg/kg/hr infusion	
Urinary retention	Replace urinary catheter prn	

young children. Postoperative respiratory depression is greatly reduced by avoiding intraoperative opioids and using prudent doses of spinal and epidural opioids.

The risk of epidural hematoma formation is small but finite. This risk can be minimized by employing reasonable safeguards. Appropriate precautions include selecting patients with normal coagulation function prior to needle placement, abandoning the regional anesthesia technique if needle placement is difficult, and delaying surgery in the event of return of blood via the needle or epidural catheter. The time interval between needle placement and heparin administration should be maximized, allowing for an interval of at least 60 minutes. Epidural catheters should be removed only after normal coagulation function has been restored following surgery.

Future studies may provide additional information regarding the dose-response relationships of regional anesthetic agents in patients undergoing cardiac surgery. Modulation of the stress response in neonates, e.g., utilizing total spinal anesthesia, warrants investigation. In addition, strategies to decrease the incidence of side effects (e.g., prophylactic antiemetic therapy) may be developed.

References

1. Weissman C: The metabolic response to stress: An overview and update. Anesthesiology 73:308–327, 1990
2. Kehlet H: Surgical stress: the role of pain and analgesia. Br J Anaesth 63:189–95, 1989
3. Anand KJS, Hansen DD, Hickey PR: Hormonal-metabolic stress responses in neonates undergoing cardiac surgery. Anesthesiology 73:661–670, 1990
4. Bromage PR, Shibata HR, Willoughby HW: Influence of prolonged epidural blockade on blood sugar and cortisol responses to operations upon the upper part of the abdomen and thorax. Surg Gynecol Obstet 132:1051–1056, 1971
5. Kirno K, Friberg P, Grzegorczyk A, et al: Thoracic epidural anesthesia during coronary artery bypass surgery: Effects on cardiac sympathetic activity, myocardial blood flow and metabolism, and central hemodynamics. Anesth Analg 79:1075–1081, 1994
6. Stenseth R, Bjella L, Berg EM, et al: Thoracic epidural analgesia in aortocoronary bypass surgery, II. Effects on the endocrine metabolic response. Acta Anaesthesiol Scand 38:834-9, 1994
7. Moore CM, Cross MH, Desborough JP, et al: Hormonal effects of thoracic extradural analgesia for cardiac surgery. Br J Anaesth 75:387-93, 1995
8. Fawcett WJ, Edwards RE, Quinn AC, et al: Thoracic epidural analgesia started after cardiopulmonary bypass. Adrenergic, car-

diovascular and respiratory sequelae. Anaesthesia 52:294-99, 1997.

9. El-Baz N, Goldin M: Continuous epidural infusion of morphine for pain relief after cardiac operations. J Thorac Cardiovasc Surg 93:878-83, 1987.

10. Rosen DA, Rosen KR, Matheny JM, et al: Maintenance of T3 levels in children undergoing cardiac surgery. Anesthesiology 87:A1069, 1997.

11. Wolf AR, Eyres RL, Laussen PC, et al: Effect of extradural analgesia on stress responses to abdominal surgery in infants. British Journal of Anaesthesia 70:654-660, 1993.

12. Liu S, Carpenter RL, Neal JM: Epidural anesthesia and analgesia: their role in postoperative outcome. Anesthesiology 82:1474–1506, 1995

13. Salomaki TE, Leppaluoto J, Laitinen JO, et al: Epidural vs. intravenous fentanyl for reducing hormonal, metabolic, and physiologic responses after thoracotomy. Anesthesiology 79:672–679, 1993

14. Fenton KN, Heinemann MK, Hickey PR, et al: Inhibition of the fetal stress response improves cardiac output and gas exchange after fetal cardiac bypass. J Thorac Cardiovasc Surg 107:1416–1422, 1994.

15. Gruber EM, Laussen PC, Casta A, et al. Stress response in infants undergoing cardiac surgery: a randomized study of fentanyl bolus, fentanyl infusion, and fentanyl-midazolam infusion. Anesth Analg 92:882-90, 2001.

16. Guinard JP, Mavrocordatos P, Chiolero R, Carpenter RL: A randomized comparison of intravenous versus lumbar and thoracic epidural fentanyl for analgesia after thoracotomy. Anesthesiology 77:1108–1115, 1992

17. Slinger P, Shennib H, Wilson S: Postthoracotomy pulmonary function: a comparison of epidural versus intravenous meperidine infusion. J Cardiothorac Vasc Anesth 9:128–134, 1995

18. Mankikan B, Cantineau JP, Berttrand M, et al: Improvement in diaphragmatic function by a thoracic extradural block after upper abdominal surgery. Anesthesiology 68:1379–1386, 1988

19. Jones SEF, Beasley JM, Macfarlane DWR, et al: Intrathecal morphine for postoperative pain relief in children. Br J Anaesth 56:137–140, 1984

20. Shayevitz JR, Merkel S, O'Kelly SW, et al: Lumbar epidural morphine infusions for children undergoing cardiac surgery. J Cardiothorac Vasc Anesth 10:217–224, 1996

21. Rosen KR, Rosen DA: Caudal epidural morphine for control of pain following open heart surgery in children. Anesthesiology 70:418–421, 1989

22. Steinbrook RA: Epidural anesthesia and gastrointestinal motility. Anesth Analg 86:837–844, 1998
23. de Leon-Casasola OA, Karabella D, Lema MJ: Bowel function recovery after radical hysterectomies: thoracic epidural bupivacaine-morphine versus intravenous patient-controlled analgesia with morphine—a pilot study. J Clin Anesth 8:87–92, 1996
24. Kock M, Blomberg S, Emanuelsson H, et al: Thoracic epidural anesthesia improves global and regional left ventricular function during stress-induced myocardial ischemia in patients with coronary artery disease. Anesth Analg 71:625–630, 1990
25. Blomberg SG: Long term home self-treatment with high thoracic epidural anesthesia in patients with severe coronary artery disease. Anesth Analg 79:413-21, 1994.
26. Blomberg S, Curelaru I, Emanuelsson H, et al: Thoracic epidural anesthesia in patients with unstable angina pectoris. Eur Heart J 10:437–444, 1989
27. Sivarajan M, Amory DW, Lindbloom LE, Schwettmann RS: Systemic and regional blood-flow changes during spinal anesthesia in the rhesus monkey. Anesthesiology 43:78–88, 1975
28. Dohi S, Naito H, Takahashi T: Age-related changes in blood pressure and duration of motor block in spinal anesthesia. Anesthesiology 50:319–323, 1979
29. Finkel JC, Boltz MG, Conran AM, et al: Hemodynamic changes during spinal anesthesia in children undergoing open heart surgery. Anesth Analg 86:S400, 1998
30. Hammer GB, Ngo K, Macario A: A retrospective examination of regional plus general anesthesia in children undergoing open heart surgery. Anesth Analg 2000; 90:1020–4.
31. Krane EJ, Tyler DC, Jacobson LE: The dose response of caudal morphine in children. Anesthesiology 71:48–52,1989.
32. Wolf AR, Hughes D, Hobbs AJ, Prys-Roberts C: Combined morphine-bupivacaine caudals for reconstructive penile surgery in children: Systemic absorption of morphine and post-operative analgesia. Anaesth Intens Care 19:17–21, 1991
33. Shapiro LA, Jedeikin RJ, Shalev D, Hoffman S: Epidural morphine analgesia in children. Anesthesiology 61:210–212, 1984.
34. Krane EJ, Jacobson LE, Lynn AM, et al: Caudal morphine for postoperative analgesia in children: A comparison with caudal bupivacaine and intravenous morphine. Anesth Analg 66:647–653, 1987
35. Chaney MA, Furry PA, Fluder EM, Slogoff S: Intrathecal morphine for coronary artery bypass grafting and early extubation. Anesth Analg 84:241–248, 1997
36. Tobias JD, Deshpande JK, Wetzell RC, et al: Postoperative analgesia: Use of intrathecal morphine in children. Clin Pediatrics 29:44–48, 1990

37. Finkel JC, Doyle JM, Conran AM, Boltz MG: A comparison of 3 intrathecal morphine doses during spinal anesthesia in children having open heart surgery. Anesthesiology 87:A1052, 1997
38. Tryba M: Epidural regional anesthesia and low molecular weight heparin: Pro (German). Anasth Intensivmed Notfallmed Schmertzther 28:179–181, 1993.
39. Vandermeulen EP, Van Aken H, Vermylen J: Anticoagulants and spinal-epidural anesthesia. Anesth Analg 79:1165–1177, 1994
40. Rao TLK, El-Etr AA: Anticoagulation following placement of epidural and subarachnoid catheters: An evaluation of neurologic sequelae. Anesthesiology 55:618–620, 1981
41. Chaney MA: Intrathecal and epidural anesthesia and analgesia for cardiac surgery. Anesth Analg 84:1211–1221, 1997
42. Mathews ET, Abrams LD: Intrathecal morphine in open heart surgery (correspondence). Lancet 2:543, 1980
43. Vanstrum GS, Bjornson KM, Ilko R: Postoperative effects of intrathecal morphine in coronary bypass surgery. Anesth Analg 67:261–67, 1988
44. Kowalewski RJ, MacAdams CL, Eagle CJ, et al: Anaesthesia for coronary bypass surgery supplemented with subarachnoid bupivacaine and morphine: A report of 18 cases. Can J Anaesth 41:1189–1195, 1994
45. Hoar PF, Hickey PF, Ullyot DJ: Systemic hypertension following myocardial revascularization: A method of treatment using epidural anesthesia. J Thorac Cardiovasc Surg 71:859–864, 1976
46. Bromage PR, Camporesi EM, Durant PAC, et al: Rostral spread of epidural morphine. Anesthesiology 56:431–436, 1982.
47. Dahlstrom B: Pharmacokinetics and pharmacodynamics of epidural and intrathecal morphine. Int Anesthesiol Clin 24:29–42, 1986.
48. Schulte-Steinberg O, Rahlfs VW: Spread of extradural analgesia following caudal injection in children. Br J Anaesth 49:1027–1034, 1982
49. Satoyoshi M, Kaniyama Y: Caudal anaesthesia for upper abdominal surgery in infants and children: A simple calculation of the volume of local anaesthesia. Acta Anaesthesiol Scand 28:57–60,1984
50. Bosenberg AT, Bland BA, Schulte-Steinberg O, et al: Thoracic epidural anesthesia via the caudal route in infants. Anesthesiology 69:265–269, 1988
51. Goodarzi M: Comparison of epidural morphine, hydromorphone and fentanyl for postoperative pain control in children undergoing orthopaedic surgery. Paed Anaes 9:419–422, 1999

Peter D. Slinger, M.D., F.R.C.P.(C)
Karen McRae, M.D.C.M., F.R.C.P.(C)

7 | Regional Anesthesia for Thoracotomy

INTRODUCTION

Respiratory complications have been the major cause of morbidity and mortality after pulmonary resection surgery. The thoracic surgical population differs in this from other adult surgical groups, where cardiac complications are the commonest cause of morbidity and mortality. Studies prior to 1990 consistently report a higher rate (15–20%) of major respiratory complications (atelectasis, pneumonia, respiratory failure) following thoracic surgery than cardiac complications (ischemia, arrhythmia) (10–15%) (1, 2). The incidence of post-thoracotomy respiratory complications has shown an overall decline in the last decade to less than 10% while the cardiac complication rate has not changed (3). This decrease in respiratory complications has led to a decrease in mortality, which is the major cause of the improvement seen in outcome following lung cancer resection seen in the past decade (see Table 7–1). It is now becoming evident that improvements in postoperative care, specifically pain management, are the major cause of this decline (4).

THE PATHOPHYSIOLOGY OF THORACOTOMY

The recovery of pulmonary function following thoracotomy is unique when compared to other types of surgical incisions (see Figure 7–1) (5). Although the loss of immediate lung mechanical force is not as severe due to the incision itself (the patients shown in Figure 7–1 did not have

Regional Anesthesia for Cardiothoracic Surgery, edited by Mark Chaney,
Lippincott Williams & Wilkins, Baltimore © 2002.

Table 7–1. Recent Trends in Perioperative Mortality following Lung Cancer Surgery

Authors	Year	Patients	Mortality (%)	Analgesic technique
Nakahara (1, 2)	1988	All risks	6.4	IV/IM
Licker (4)	1993	All risks	4.8	IV/IM/LEA
Cerfolio (3)	1996	High risk	2.4	LEA/TEA
Licker (4)	1997	All risks	2.1	TEA

IV= intravenous, IM= intramuscular, LEA= lumbar epidural analgesia, TEA= thoracic epidural analgesia

resection of lung tissue), compared to upper abdominal surgery, the recovery is delayed in the first 3 days during the time period when pulmonary function is recovering after other types of surgery. It is during this plateau of recovery from days 1–3 that the majority of major post-thoracotomy pulmonary complications occur. The early postoperative loss of lung function will depend on the type of thoracotomy incision (6) and is least for anterolateral or muscle-sparing incisions compared to standard posterolateral thoracotomies and is worst with the bilateral trans-sternal "clamshell " incisions.

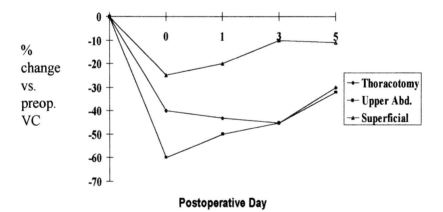

Postoperative Day

FIGURE 7–1. The recovery of mechanical lung function expressed as percent of preoperative vital capacity (VC) following various types of surgical incisions over the first 5 days following surgery (thoracotomy patients did not have resection of lung tissue). Note that although the immediate respiratory impairment is most severe following upper abdominal surgery, there is a trend to return of function that begins on the first postoperative day. Recovery of mechanical respiratory function is delayed for 3 days following thoracotomy. Based on the data of Ali et al. (5).

TABLE 7–2. Post-thoracotomy Pain Pathways

Pain source	Afferent conduction
Incision	Intercostal nerves (4–6)
Chest drains	Intercostal nerves (5–8)
Mediastinal pleura	Vagus nerve
Central diaphragmatic pleura	Phrenic nerve
Ipsilateral shoulder	Brachial plexus (?)

There are multiple sensory afferents that transmit nociceptive stimuli following thoracotomy (see Table 7–2). It is impossible to imagine that any one technique or medication can cover all these sources of pain. The basis of post-thoracotomy analgesia must be multimodal therapy, and regional anesthesia forms an essential part of this plan (see Table 7–3).There is no one analgesic method that is applicable in all situations. The optimal choice for an individual patient will depend on patient factors (contraindications, preferences), surgical factors (type of incision), and system factors (available equipment, monitoring, nursing support). The ideal post-thoracotomy analgesic technique will include three classes of drugs: opioids, nonsteroidal anti-inflammatory drugs (NSAIDs), and local anesthetics. These three are all evidence-based choices. Other methods such as cryoanalgesia and transcutaneous electrical nerve stimulation will also be mentioned.

SYSTEMIC ANALGESIA

Opioids

Systemic opioids alone are effective in controlling background pain, but the acute pain component associated with coughing or movement requires plasma levels that are associated with sedation and hypoventilation in most patients (7). Even when administered by patient-controlled devices, pain control is generally poor after thoracotomy (8), and patients have interrupted sleep patterns when serum opioid levels fall below the therapeutic range.

TABLE 7–3. Multimodal Post-thoracotomy Analgesia

Regional anesthesia: infiltration, intercostal, intrapleural, extrapleural, epidural
Opioids: oral, transdermal, subcutaneous, intramuscular, intravenous, epidural, spinal
Nonsteroidal anti—inflammatory drugs (NSAIDs): oral, rectal, intravenous
Other drugs/modalities: Ketamine, alpha2-agonists, transcutaneous electrical nerve stimulation (TENS), cryoanalgesia

Nonsteroidal Anti-inflammatory Drugs (NSAIDs)

NSAIDs can reduce opioid consumption >30% following thoracotomy (9) and are particularly useful treating the ipsilateral shoulder pain that is often present postoperatively. This pain seems to be musculoskeletal in origin and is poorly contolled with epidural analgesia (there is no consensus on the origin of this pain, which has also been attributed to phrenic nerve irritation and a variety of other sources). NSAIDs act through reversible inhibition of cyclo-oxygenase, which has anti-inflammatory and analgesic effects but can also be associated with decreased platelet function, gastric erosions, increased bronchial reactivity, and decreased renal function. Newer NSAIDs such as celecoxib and meloxicam have a lower tendency to inhibit the homeostatic cycloxygenase isoenzyme (COX-1) and are more potent inhibitors of the anti-inflammatory (COX-2) isoenzyme. They are associated with less adverse gastrointestinal side effects and less platelet inhibition. The renal safety profile seems equivalent to other NSAIDs(10).

Ketamine

In low doses, ketamine may produce analgesia via noncompetitive blockade of N-methyl-D-aspartate (NMDA) receptors(11). Low dose intramuscular (IM) ketamine (1mg/kg) is equivalent to the same dose of IM meperidine and causes less respiratory depression(12). Ketamine can also be administered as a low dose IV infusion and may be useful in patients who are refractory to other therapies or where there is a contraindication to more common techniques(13). The possibility of psychomimetic effects with ketamine is always a concern but is rarely seen with subanesthetic doses.

REGIONAL TECHNIQUES

Intercostal Blocks

Blocks of the intercostal nerves supplying the dermatomes of the surgical incision are an effective adjunct to methods of post-thoracotomy analgesia. These can be done percutaneously or under direct vision when the chest is open. The duration of analgesia is transient and the blocks will need to be repeated to have any useful effect on postoperative lung function(14). Indwelling intercostal catheters are an option (15) and can be used for boluses or infusions, but they can be difficult to position reliably percutaneously and they are difficult to secure in place.

The intercostal nerves lie consistently between the same anatomical planes, deep to the internal intercostal muscle and superficial to the endothoracic fascia, which is in turn superficial to the parietal pleura. Local anesthetic deposited in the correct plane will reliably block the nerve even though the course of the nerve often lies in the middle or lower portion of the intercostal space and is not confined to the subcostal groove as classically described(16). Small boluses (< 5 ml) will tend to remain at the site of injection. Larger boluses can produce multiple level intercostal blockade by extension medially to the paravertebral space or by direct extrapleural extension superior and inferior to adjacent intercostal spaces(17). Systemic uptake of local anesthetic is rapid from the intercostal space compared to other sites of regional anesthesia and doses must be adjusted with the possibility of systemic toxicity in mind(14).

It is important to fully understand the anatomy of the intercostal nerve to appreciate the potential usefulness and limitations of intercostal nerve blockade. Note in Figure 7–2 that there are three main sen-

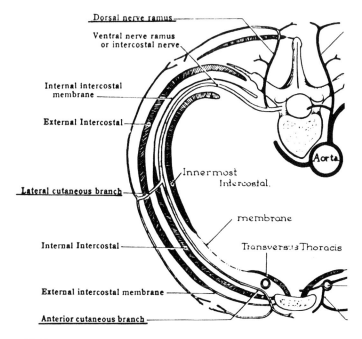

FIGURE 7–2.   Diagram of an intercostal nerve. Note the location of the three cutaneous branches: anterior, lateral, and posterior, which are derived from the dorsal nerve ramus. An intercostal block must be placed at or posterior to the posterior axillary line to be certain to block the lateral branch. The posterior branch, which will supply the innervation for the posterior end of a traditional posterolateral thoracotomy incision cannot be blocked with an intercostal block (from *Grant's Atlas of Anatomy*, Baltimore: Lippincott Williams & Wilkins, 1962, with permission).

sory branches, the posterior, lateral, and anterior cutaneous nerves. It is not possible to anesthetize the posterior branch with an intercostal block. Thus, intercostal blocks are less useful for the traditional posterolateral thoracotomy incision than they are for the lateral or anterolateral incisions now favored by some surgeons. Also, intercostal blocks are useful for chest-drain incision pain and can be used for awake thoracoscopy. It is important that the intercostal nerve is blocked at or posterior to the posterior axillary line so that the lateral cutaneous branch can be reliably anesthetized. This usually requires turning a supine patient to a lateral or semilateral position to place the block.

Cryoanalgesia

Application of a $-60°C$ probe to the exposed intercostal nerves in the open thorax intraoperatively produces an intercostal block that can persist for up to 6 months. This technique can be moderately efficient to decrease postoperative pain but is associated with an incidence of chronic neuralgia that has led many centers to abandon the procedure(18, 19). It is not certain that the incidence of long-term neuralgia exceeds that seen from the thoracotomy incision itself. One study of long-term postoperative pain in patients who had not received cryoanalgesia found that >50% of patients reported pain at the incision for more than 1 year following thoracotomy(20). A randomized study found the pain relief from cryoanalgesia inferior to thoracic epidural fentanyl(21). Open intercostal nerve phenol injections have been also used for post-thoracotomy pain with results similar to cryoanalgesia(22).

Intrapleural Analgesia

Post-thoracotomy pain relief has been attempted by injection/infusion of local anesthetics directly into the pleural cavity. This same technique is called "intrapleural" and "interpleural" by different authors. Initial reports of this technique were favorable(23). Intrapleural local anesthetics produce a multilevel intercostal block, and some centers have been able to obtain satisfactory analgesia with this method (24), although the volumes of local anesthetics required are large (e.g., 7 ml/hr of 0.5% bupivacaine). However, the analgesia is extremely dependent on patient position, infusion volume, and the type of surgery. In spite of occasional successes, most clinicians have not found the reliability of intrapleural techniques adequate to justify their use on a routine basis (25, 26).

Paravertebral Block

This technique of analgesia, first described in the early 1900s, has undergone a recent revival of interest as a method of routine post-thoracotomy analgesia(27). A catheter can be placed in the thoracic paravertebral space either under direct vision intraoperatively (see Figure 7–3) or percutaneously. Unfortunately, this block is also called "extrapleural " or "intercostal" by different authors, so there tends to be some

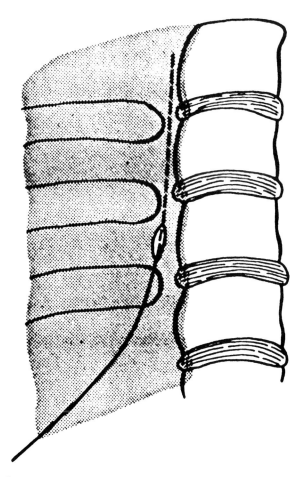

FIGURE 7–3a.   One method of placement of a paravertebral catheter intraoperatively. The parietal pleura (stippled) is raised from the posterior chest wall. An epidural catheter is passed into the paravertebaral space through a small defect created in the extrapleural (endothoracic) fascia. The proximal end of the catheter is then brought out of the chest through a separate needle puncture in an intercostal space near the chest drains (from Berrisford and Sabanathan (28), with permission).

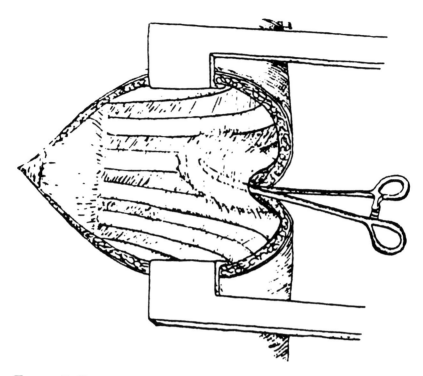

FIGURE 7–3b. An alternative method of placement of a paravertaebral catheter is to create an extrapleural pocket at the posterior end of the surgical incision. The catheter is introduced pecutaneously into this pocket under direct vision by a needle placed through an intercostal space directly into the pocket. This "extrapleural" block may function more as a multilevel intercostal block if the pocket is not developed medially to the paravertebral space. (from Watson et al. (29), with permission).

confusion in the literature. As can be seen in Figure 7–3 there is no agreement on the best position of these catheters, and some may be more truly intercostal than paravertebral depending on how they are placed(28, 29). The most clinically useful technique is to have the surgeon place the catheter with the chest open just prior to closure. Some variation in the efficacy of the block may depend on whether the catheter is placed deep (preferred) or superficial to the endothoracic fascia(30).

An initial bolus of local anesthetic (e.g.,10–20 ml bupivacaine, 0.25–0.5%) is administered with the chest open to assure that there is adequate rostral-caudal spread in the paravertebral space with minimal leakage into the interpleural space. Then an infusion of local anesthetic (5–8 ml/hr) is continued for 3 to 5 days postoperatively. Bupivacaine with/without epinephrine (5 μg/ml) and lidocaine with/without epinephrine are used in different centers. Paravertebral local anesthetics

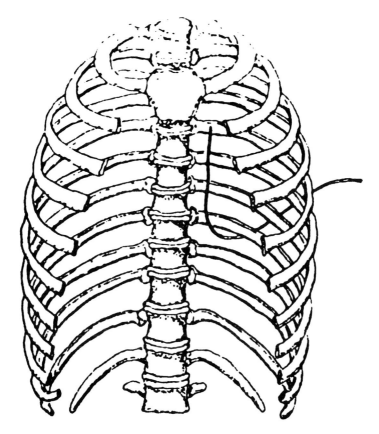

FIGURE 7–3c.   The optimal final position of a paravertebral catheter. (from
Watson et al. (29) with permission).

provide a reliable multilevel intercostal nerve blockade (usually 3–5 de-
matomes (31)) that tends to be unilateral with a low tendency to spread
to the epidural space.

Clinically, the analgesia is comparable to that from epidural local
anesthetics. No regional technique (intercostal, paravertebral, or epidural)
provides sufficient analgesia when used alone with only local anesthet-
ics(32). Paravertebral bupivacaine infusions in combination with NSAIDs
and systemic opioids offer a reasonable alternative to epidural techniques in children (33) or patients with contraindications to neuraxial
blockade. However, using common theraputic doses (e.g., 0.1 ml/kg/hr
of bupivacaine, 0.5%) serum bupivacaine levels can approach toxic levels
by 4 days(34).

Paravertebral catheters can be placed percutaneously for thoracic
analgesia in patients who do not have an open chest(27). Indications for

this technique do not arise commonly in clinical practice but may occur in chest trauma with multiple rib fractures when there is a contraindication to neuraxial analgesia (e.g., concurrent spinal trauma or coagulopathy). Paravertebral catheters can also be placed in thoracoscopy patients using video guidance for unilateral or bilateral thoracoscopic surgery(35).

Transcutaneous Electrical Nerve Stimulation (TENS)

TENS may be useful when pain is mild to moderate but is ineffective when pain is severe(36). At best, it may decrease opioid requirements and limit the side effects of nausea and vomiting(37, 38).

Spinal Analgesia

The application of opioids or local anesthetics to the neuraxis for analgesia is an anesthetic practice that has evolved continuously over the past 115 years since the first documented use of spinal cocaine by Corning (39). High spinal anesthesia combined with general anesthesia was a thoracic anesthesia technique popular in the 1930s. This was done in spontaneously breathing patients. However, the introduction of the routine use of positive pressure ventilation to assure intraoperative gas exchange and the hemodynamic instability associated with high spinals subsequently made this an unattractive technique. In the 1980s, the use of spinal techniques with opioids for postoperative pain combined with general anesthesia experienced a revival. Adequate post-thoracotomy analgesia for 12 to 24 hours can be obtained from a single pre- or intraoperative lumbar spinal injection of a hydophilic opioid such as morphine(40). This technique has not received widespread application due to the fact that it is a single bolus method that can have unpredictable side effects, particularly delayed respiratory depression. Also, the analgesia wears off during the 24- 72-hour postoperative period when the patients most need pain relief as they begin to mobilize. Repeated intrathecal injections and the use of spinal catheters are not acceptable to most clinicians.

In certain select situations there may be some potential benefits of this technique over thoracic epidural analgesia. Many anesthesiologists feel comfortable doing a lumbar spinal puncture in anesthetized patients, so there may be some indication for patients who wish neuraxial analgesia but prefer it done during general anesthesia. Some anesthesiologists feel that there is less risk of an epidural hematoma from a spinal versus an epidural injection. Also, there may be an occasional patient where for technical reasons, such as previous thoracic spine surgery, it is not possible to place a thoracic epidural. However, in our practice most of these patients now receive paravertebral analgesia. Some of the early reports of respiratory depression from spinal analgesia may relate to the use of excessive doses of morphine ($> 10 \mu g/kg$) while doses of 5 to $7\mu g/kg$ are often adequate.

Epidural Analgesia

A meta-analysis of respiratory complications following various types of surgery has shown that only epidural techniques reduce the incidence of respiratory complications (41).There were not enough comparative studies to differentiate between lumbar epidural analgesia (LEA) and thoracic epidural analgesia (TEA). This study also showed that the only predictive test for improved respiratory outcome was decreased pain with motion. Introduced into routine clinical practice in the 1980s (42), LEA has gradually been replaced by TEA in the 1990s. In a survey of Australian hospitals published in 1997, Cook and Riley (43) reported that 10 of 12 hospitals performing >100 thoracotomies/year used epidurals as their routine method of postoperative analgesia. In this survey, epidurals were routinely placed at mid-thoracic levels (>90%), used local anesthetic plus opioid mixtures (>95%), used continuous infusions (100%), and were continued for 3 or more days postoperatively (>80%). Another meta-analysis of postoperative outcome has shown that thoracic but not lumbar epidurals decrease mortality(44). However, this study was not limited to thoracic surgery.

The evolution of routine thoracic epidural infusion analgesia has been delayed pending advances in technology and knowledge. The technology required was the development of portable, safe, and reliable infusion pumps that did not delay postoperative ambulation. The knowledge required was in four areas.

First, the importance of the synergy between local anesthetics and opioids for segmental thoracic analgesia has only been recently documented (45). The addition of an opioid versus placebo to a thoracic epidural bupivacaine infusion in a double-blind study gave better analgesia at rest during the first 24 hours postoperatively and better analgesia with movement for 72 hours (46). Similarly, adding bupivacaine versus placebo to an epidural opioid infusion led to opioid sparing and better analgesia during physiotherapy (47, 48).

Second, the concern for patient risks due to postoperative thoracic epidural analgesia has delayed widespread acceptance. The real and well-documented risks of respiratory depression (49) and hemodynamic instability (50) seem to have been largely due to the use of bolus epidural injections. The use of epidural infusions now has an excellent record for patient safety when used on routine postoperative surgical wards (51, 52). The risk of accidental direct spinal cord trauma from thoracic epidural needles and catheters has slowed the adoption of this technique by many anesthesiologists. A recent study of >4,000 TEA placements in a German teaching hospital (53) documented no permanent neurologic sequellae and a 1% incidence of accidental dural puncture, which was less than the expected risk of dural puncture for lumbar epidurals. The specialty of anesthesia is becoming more accustomed to the safety of the technique.

Third, many anesthesiologists believe that thoracic epidural catheter placement is a difficult technique. The study by Giebler et al. (53) demonstrated a 1% incidence of technical failure, a success rate that rivals any other form of regional blockade.

Finally, many anesthesiologists are not comfortable with the technique, not having had adequate exposure during their training. Until these developments of the past 10 years made TEA a useful adjunct for routine thoracic anesthesia, there was little indication to train residents in the technique except for those with an interest in chronic pain therapy. Now, progressive training programs feel it is a vital tool for residents to have mastered by the end of their training. For those already in practice, workshops are offered by both national and regional anesthesia societies. However, the technique is similar enough to lumbar epidural catheter placement that it is quite feasible to learn "on the job" with the guidance of a colleague.

The Pharmacology of Synergy

Recent research has begun to shed some light on the physiology and pharmacology that underlie the synergy between local anesthetics and opioids to produce segmental epidural analgesia (54). In a double-blind randomized study, Hansdottir et al. (48) compared epidural infusions of lumbar sufentanil, thoracic sufentanil, and thoracic sufentanil plus bupivacaine (S+B) for post-thoracotomy analgesia (see Figure 7–4). Infusions were titrated for equianalgesia at rest. Thoracic sufentanil plus bupivacaine provided significantly better analgesia with movement and less sedation than the other infusions. Although sufentanil dosages and serum levels were significantly lower in the combined (S+B) group than in the other two groups, lumbar cerebropspinal fluid (CSF) levels of sufentanil at 24 and 48 hours were higher in the combined group than in the thoracic sufentanil group. This suggests that local anesthetics facilitate the entry of opioid from the epidural space into the CSF.

Also, in an animal study by Tejwani et al. (55), the binding of morphine to spinal K-receptors was significantly augmented in the presence of local anesthetics (see Figure 7–5). The authors theorize that local

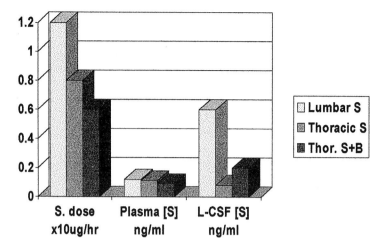

FIGURE 7–4. Differences in the pharmacology of post-thoractomy epidural infusions of lumbar sufentanil (Lumbar S), thoracic sufentanil (Thoracic S) and thoracic sufentanil plus bupivacaine (Thor. S + B). Thoracic S + B produced significantly superior analgesia with movement with lower total sufentanil dosage (S. dose) and lower plasma levels (Plasma [S]) than the other two techniques. Note that in spite of lower dosage, thoracic S + B patients had higher mean lumbar cerebrospinal fluid (CSF) sufentanil levels than the thoracic sufentanil group measured by separate lumbar punctures at 24 and 48 hours postoperatively. This suggests a pharmacokinetic mechanism with local anesthetics that facilitates transfer of epidural opioid into the CSF (from Slinger (54), with permission).

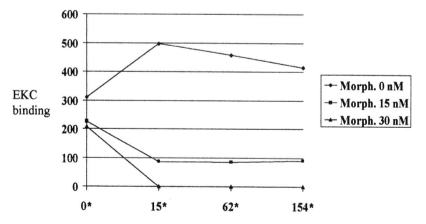

FIGURE 7–5. The effects of spinal morphine and bupivacaine on the binding of EKC (a K-ligand) to opioid receptors in the spinal cord of rats. Bupivacaine produced a tenfold increase in morphine induced antinociception. This correlated with increased displacement of EKC from spinal K-receptors in the presence of both morphine and bupivacaine (i.e., increased affinity of morphine for the opioid receptors). This synergy occurred at the lowest concentration of bupivacaine studied and was not augmented by increasing the bupivacaine dosage (from Slinger (54), with permission).

anesthetics may cause a conformational change in the K-receptor that facilitates opioid binding. Particularly of note is that this synergy occurred at the lowest doses of local anesthetic studied and was not significantly increased as the local anesthetic concentration was increased. This suggests that the clinically important synergy between local anesthetics and opioids to produce segmental epidural analgesia may be effective at very low doses of local anesthetic, which will avoid the well-known side effects of sympathetic blockade.

Respiratory Effects of TEA

It was initially theorized that TEA could diminish the diaphragmatic inhibition that is known to occur after thoracotomy(56). Such disinhibition was shown for TEA after upper abdominal surgery (57). Indeed, a post-thoracotomy animal model demonstrated similar disinhibition (58). However, a post-thoracotomy human study of patients with moderate chronic obstructive pulmonary disease (COPD) failed to show any improvement of diaphragmatic contractility by TEA, even though respiratory function (tidal volume) was improved (59). This is not easy to explain but it may be similar to the concept of increasing cardiac output without increasing myocardial contractility by changing loading conditions for the ventricle. The diaphragm inserts on the chest wall, and by decreasing chest splinting, the diaphragm may be returned to a mechanically more efficient position on its force-length (Starling) contraction curve without affecting its actual contractility.

It has been shown in volunteers that a thoracic level of epidural blockade increases FRC.[60] This increase is largely due to an increase in thoracic gas volume caused by a fall in the resting level of the diaphragm without a fall in tidal volume. This contradicts earlier studies which found no change in functional reserve capacity (FRC) with TEA(61). The different results are probably related to the more advanced methodology of the recent work. FRC is considered the most important determinant of oxygenation in the postoperative period (62).

There has been a concern that the nerve block produced by thoracic epidural local anesthetic may have a deleterious effect on respiratory function in patients with severe COPD. While the possibility still exists that a thoracic motor block may impair respiratory function, there are clearly no negative effects from the sensory block associated with typical analgesic doses of local anesthetic. Gruber et al. (63) studied a group of patients with severe COPD (mean FEV_1 = 27% predicted) and found that the sensory block from 10 to 12 ml of 0.25% bupivacaine (mean number of blocked segments= 8) produced a slight but significant increase in tidal volume and decrease in lung resistance without any significant effect on other measures of pulmonary mechanics.

Although it is possible to deliver an opioid to the spinal cord receptors via a lumbar catheter in adequate amounts for analgesia, the beneficial synergistic effects of local anesthetics on respiratory mechanics require a thoracic catheter. Improvement in respiratory function with combined local anesthetic and opioid TEA has been confirmed in post-thoracotomy clinical studies (45, 48).

Cardiovascular Effects of TEA

The leading cardiovascular cause of morbidity and mortality after thoracic surgery is arrhythmias, particularly atrial fibrillation, which occurs in approximately 15% of patients following lung resection surgery (64). In-hospital mortality is increased from 2% to 17% in those post-thoracotomy patients who develop arrhythmias. Arrhythmias also correlate with poor long-term outcome. Mean survival in patients 18 months following lung resection for cancer was decreased to 10% in patients who had early postoperative arrhythmias versus 57% in those without arrhythmias (65).

The cause of post-thoracotomy arrhythmias is due to the interaction of two factors: right heart strain and increased sympathetic nervous system stimulation(66). In theory, TEA can decrease both of these causes of arrhythmia. In animal models of ischemia, TEA has been shown to decrease arrhythmias by decreasing sympathetic tone. In a recent study of prophylactic oxygen administration to decrease post-thoracotomy arrhythmias, Backlund et al. (67) found no clinically significant episodes of postoperative atrial fibrillation in their control group (those patients who received supplemental oxygen for only the first 24 hours). This compares with an incidence of 30% in a similar control group from a previous study by the same research group (68). The major difference between the two control groups was that the recent group received TEA and the previous group did not. No statistical conclusions can be reached comparing the two groups but the data suggest that the TEA group had lower right-heart pressures.

Perioperative myocardial ischemia occurs in approximately 5% of post-thoracotomy patients, which is what would be expected for any major surgery in a patient population of this age with a high incidence of smoking. The benefits of TEA as a treatment for myocardial ischemia are well known (69). The sympathetic blockade from TEA in patients with coronary artery disease decreases both myocardial oxygen demand and supply but has no net effect on echocardiographic segmental wall motion, which is the most sensitive indicator of ischemia (70). This is in contrast to the effects of LEA, which can induce segmental wall motion abnormalities in patients with known coronary artery disease as myocardial oxygen supply is decreased but demand is not affected (71).

There has been a concern that thoracic sympathetic blockade from local anesthetics can cause problematic hypotension in postoperative patients. However, with the use of synergistic combinations of local anesthetics and opioids, and limiting the total dose of local anesthetics, this problem can be avoided. Moniche et al. (52) in a study of upper abdominal surgery found that TEA infusions of bupivacaine 0.25% and morphine 0.05 mg/ml at a mean rate of 4 ml/hour produced superior analgesia to intravenous/intramuscular morphine, and there were no differences between groups in blood pressures at rest, standing, or walking. The only significant hemodynamic difference between groups was a slightly lower heart rate in the TEA group.

In patients with advanced pulmonary disease, the effects of thoracic sympathetic blockade are a concern because of potential changes in the balance between the pulmonary and systemic vascular resistances. In one case report of a patient with primary pulmonary hypertension, TEA produced a favorable effect on this balance, reducing the pulmonary artery pressure and pulmonary vascular resistance more than the systemic pressure and vascular resistance (72).

Choice of Drugs for TEA

There is no one recipe for TEA that is best in all clinical situations and it is best to be familiar with a variety of regimes and choose one that is appropriate to the individual clinical scenario and change as needed depending on the patient's tolerance and side effects. As can be seen in Figure 7–6, sensory block tends to spread more caudally when the injection is at a high thoracic level and more rostrally from a low thoracic injection (73). Ideally, the thoracic epidural catheter placement site should be as close as possible to the dermatomal level of the mid-point of the incision(s), since it is not possible to know for certain whether a catheter will tend to go higher or lower in the thoracic epidural space. In one study, even when it was attempted to have the catheters migrate rostrally in the thoracic epidural space by directing the bevel of Tuohy needle in that direction, only 9 of 22 catheters went in the intended direction (74).

When there is more than one incision (e.g., esophagogastrectomy via combined thoracotomy and laprarotomy or for thoracoscopic surgery) it is preferrable to use a hydrophilic opioid (morphine or hydromorphone) that will spread to cover more dermatomes (75). Pruritis and nausea seem to occur more with the hydophilic opioids. Systemic absorption effects (sedation) seem to be more common with the lipophilic opioids, particularly after several days of infusion.

The most commonly used local anesthetic is bupivacaine in concentrations from 0.05 to 0.25%, depending on the patient and volume. Ropivacaine or lidocaine in comparable strengths can also be used. Local

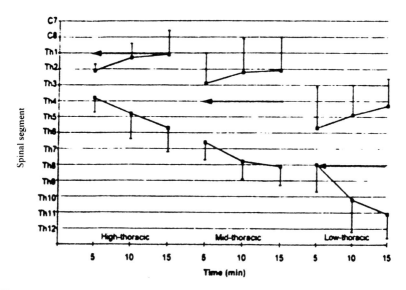

FIGURE 7–6. Extension of the sensory blockade tested by pinprick vs. time after administration of 6 ml of lidocaine 1% in the high (C2-T7), mid (T2-T4), or low thoracic epidural space. Data represent the mean +/– SD bars. Arrows indicate the level of the epidural puncture. Note that for mid or high thoracic injections the spread of the block is more caudal than rostral (from Visser et al. (73), with permission).

anesthetic dose can be decreased as needed for cardiovascular side effects (hypotension). The inclusion of epinephrine (2 μg/ml) in the epidural infusion clearly augments the analgesia produced by an opioid/local anesthetic mixture. It is not clear at present whether epinephrine is synergistic or merely additive to the other drugs (76). Nor is it certain the side effects can be reduced by the addition of epinephrine.

A sample analgesic protocol for a 60-year-old 70-kg patient with normal renal function having a thoracotomy at our institution is presented in Table 7–4. Dose ranges and alternatives are indicated in parentheses. Dosages would be decreased in smaller and older patients.

Epidural Placement: Awake versus Anesthetized

There is no international consensus on whether it is optimal practice to place a thoracic epidural catheter before or after induction of general anesthesia. Points in favor of placement postinduction include better patient comfort, the fact that active patient cooperation is not necessary, and convenience. A survey of anesthetic practice in the United Kingdom published in 1998 reported that 60% of practitioners "most often" place a thoracic epidural after induction of anesthesia (77).

TABLE 7–4. Sample Analgesic Protocol

Patient

60-year-old male, thoracotomy incision at T5, normal renal function (potential dose ranges or alternative drug choices for this patient in brackets)

Preoperatively

Heparin 5000 U subcut. 2 hr before (1 hr after) epidural placement

Intraoperatively

1. Thoracic epidural catheter placed prior to induction at T4-T5 (range T3-T7)
2. Test dose lidocaine 2% 3 cc (2–4 cc), test sensory level at 5 min
3. Following induction of anesthesia, during the period of chest incision, a bolus of fentanyl 10 μg/ml plus bupivacaine 0.2% in 2 cc increments as tolerated to a maximum total dose 10 cc (4–10 cc) guided by BP
4. Minimal systemic opioids following induction and intubation
5. Ketorolac 30 mg IV (15–30 mg) before chest closure
6. Begin postoperative analgesic epidural infusion (see below) intraoperatively 1–2 hr after induction with p.r.n. boluses of epidural solution (2–3 ml) during chest closure guided by BP

Postoperatively

1. Patient-controlled epidural analgesia (PCEA) with fixed infusion rate and p.r.n. boluses.
   TEA Infusion: Bupivacaine 0.1% (0.1–.05%) plus hydromorphone 15 μg/ml*(or morphine 50 μg/ml, or fentanyl 4 μg/ml) at 6 ml/hr (3–8 ml/hr) with boluses 3 ml (2–4 ml) q 20 min p.r.n., 4 hr max. dose limit 40 ml
2. Ketorolac 15–30 mg IV q 12 hr (rectal indomethacin 50–100 mg q 12 h) × 48 hr
3. Famotidine 10 mg IV q 12 hr × 48 hr

Monitoring on ward

Recovery room 0–2 hr, "step-down" monitored ward bed 2–24 hr, then regular ward bed > 24 hr
1. Activity: check postural blood pressure, pulse, and sensory/motor block before getting up
2. Respiratory rate and sedation scale q 1 hr for 24 hr then q 2 hr if infusion rate not increased
3. Pulse, BP q 4 hr
4. Sensory/motor block q 4 hr for 24 hr then q 8 hr if infusion rate not increased
5. Notify Acute Pain Service for :
   i)   Inadequate pain control
   ii) BP systolic <90, pulse <50, respiratory rate <10
   iii) Sedation score of 3 (somnolent, difficult to arouse)
   iv) Increasing sensory or motor block

Discontinue Epidural

Stop infusion at 72 hr (unless chest drains still in place) and observe pain control with oral opioid/anti-inflammatory. Remove catheter after satisfactory mobilization with oral analgesics.

*Opioid is discontinued in epidural solution for refractory pruritis, sedation, or other opioid side effects and the infusion is changed to Ropivacaine 0.2% with similar PCEA infusion/bolus dosing.

In contrast, a North American review of this question in the April 2001 American Society of Anesthesiologists Newsletter concluded " . . . the safety of regional anesthesia performed on anesthetized pediatric patients is not readily applicable to adults. Needle and catheter placement at the lumbar level only appears to be safe. However, techniques performed above the termination of the cord or injection of local anesthetics, which have the potential for neurotoxicity, should be avoided" (78).

Our practice at present is to routinely place epidural catheters prior to induction. Only in very exceptional circumstances (e.g., a mentally handicapped adult with consent of the guardian) and with full discussion of the risks, do we place an epidural in an anesthetized patient, and in those cases we do not administer local anesthetics until the patient regains consciousness. This choice of awake placement is in part due to medicolegal concerns but more due to our preference to be able to test the catheter and ensure a working thoracic epidural block prior to induction.

MANAGEMENT OF OPIOID-TOLERANT PATIENTS

The opioid-tolerant patient requiring thoracic surgery presents a significant challenge. Postoperative analgesia requires careful planning and frequent reassessment. Patients may be using physician prescribed opioids for pain related to their thoracic pathology or other chronic pain syndromes. Active abusers of narcotics or those in a rehabilitation program, receiving daily methadone, also are included in this group. Whenever possible, patients should take their regular analgesic or methadone preoperatively, otherwise substitute opioids must be provided.

Opioid tolerance occurs as a result of loss of active receptor sites from chronic exposure to agonist. Both a decreased number of receptors and desensitization to agonist binding are implicated (79). Clinically, the opioid doses required to produce adequate postoperative analgesia are increased.

A multimodal analgesic regimen including the use of NSAIDs and regional analgesia is optimal. A choice must be made regarding the distribution of increased opioid delivery either systemically or through an epidural catheter. Increased narcotic may be provided in the epidural solution, or standard narcotic concentrations may be used in the epidural solution with additional systemic narcotic. DeLeon-Casasola reports higher epidural doses of opioid are able to curtail the appearance of narcotic withdrawl in most patients (79). More frequently in our practice, the patient receives a standard or slightly increased concentration of opioid in the epidural infusion and additional systemic opioid to minimize the occurrence of withdrawl. A convenient way to provide drug delivery in patients not immediately able to take oral medication is in the form of a transdermal fentanyl patch. Systemic narcotic can alternately be provided as a continuous intravenous infusion or in oral format.

Patient-controlled analgesic techniques are often difficult to manage in these patients, and they may be best managed with fixed dosage regimens that are modified as needed. Ultimately, after dose titration, the patient may be receiving both increased epidural opioid and greater than preoperative doses of systemic opioid, without significant side effects. DeLeon-Casasola has documented a number of patients in whom epidural bupivicaine-morphine analgesia was inadequate who responded to a switch to bupivicaine-sufentanil (80).

Patients in drug rehabilitation programs with methadone may be very reluctant to modify their methadone dose perioperatively having struggled to establish a stable dose in the past. They frequently can take their full methadone dose throughout the perioperative period, in addition to increased epidural opioid dosing, without significant side effects.

Continuous peripheral nerve blockade such as using a paravertebral, or intercostal catheter can provide adjunctive analgesia, but these are not a route for opioid delivery and increased doses of systemic opioid must be delivered.

Supplemental therapies to be considered for these patients include adding epinephrine, 5 µg/ml, to the epidural infusion solution and the addition of low dose continuous intravenous ketamine infusions (81). All opioid tolerant patients require frequent adjustment of analgesic doses. Despite this, pain scores of 2 to –4 out of 10 with movement are often the lowest achieved. Opioid-tolerant patients' increased analgesic requirements are for a longer duration postoperatively than the usual need for analgesia in the opioid naïve.

THORACIC EPIDURAL AS PRIMARY ANESTHESIA FOR SURGERY

Several recent reports have described the use of thoracic epidurals as the primary anesthetic in conscious patients undergoing thoracic surgical procedures. Mukaida et al. (82) described four cases of high-risk patients undergoing video-assisted thoracoscopic surgery with thoracic epidural anesthesia. Three patients had severe emphysema with bilateral bullae and recurrent pneumothoraces and the fourth patient had pulmonary fibrosis with a left pneumothorax. Williams and Kay (83) reported using a combination of thoracic epidural and local infiltration of the incision site for thoracoscopy, rib resection, and minithoracotomy in an elderly patient who required a thoracic drainage procedure for a bronchopleural fistula 2 weeks post-right pneumonectomy. This technique was then continued as thoracic epidural analgesia for 3 days postoperatively. It is not clear if the addition of local infiltration of the incision was strictly necessary in these cases.

Intrathoracic diagnostic and minor therapeutic procedures have long been possible in awake patients with a combination of intercostal blocks and sedation. The use of thoracic epidurals is a logical progression of regional anesthesia for some of these cases and will undoubtedly become more frequent in the future. One advantage for these procedures of thoracic epidural versus intercostal blocks is that an epidural can block the sympathetic afferents from the perihilar plexes that trigger the cough reflex with manipulation of the hilum. However, the hilum also has vagal innervation, which will not be blocked. Also unblocked will be the mediastinal pleura and the central portion of the pleural surface of the diaphragm (see Table 7–2). Thus, when choosing to use a thoracic epidural as the main intraoperative anesthetic technique, it is important to have a clear understanding of how extensive the surgical procedure will be and which afferents need to be blocked. Problems with potential soiling of the nonoperative lung or the difficulty of converting to a general anesthetic in the lateral position if needed must always be kept in mind.

OUTCOME

Since optimal post-thoracotomy analgesia should be multimodal, and since regional analgesia is one component of multimodal pain control, is has not been possible to pick out one type of regional technique and show that it clearly improves outcome. There may never be a definitive randomized controlled double-blinded trial that clearly shows whether thoracic epidurals or any other single type of regional therapy affects outcome.

Improvements in postoperative analgesia, specifically the use of epidurals have permitted surgeons to operate on high-risk patients with improved outcomes. Cerfoilo et al. (3) reported in 1996 on a series of 85 lung resection patients who were felt to be at high-risk because of borderline pulmonary function (mean predicted postoperative $FEV_1 = 34\%$). The perioperative mortality was 2.4% (previously, a very acceptable figure in normal-risk patients) and the only deaths were cardiac in origin.

Thoracic epidurals have permitted anesthesiologists to extubate patients earlier after major intrathoracic surgery (84) and have allowed for a shift to a patient care pathway where post-thoracotomy patients can be transferred to a ward bed postoperatively without the need for a mandatory period in the intensive care unit.

One convincing piece of evidence for the effect that thoracic epidurals may have on outcome is from a study by Licker et al. (4) in 1999.

They reported retrospectively on the morbidity and mortality at their hospital following pulmonary resection for lung cancer in the period 1990–1997. At the mid-point of the study period, the routine use of thoracic epidurals with local anesthetic and opioid was introduced. The mortality significantly decreased in the second period (1994–1997 = 2.1%) versus the earlier period (1990–1993 = 4.8%). Of particular note is that the major causes of mortality shifted from respiratory causes in the early 1990s to cardiac causes in the later 1990s. If one were to argue that the improvements in outcome were due to advances in overall medical care, then it would be expected that there would be a uniform decline in morbidity and mortality from all causes. Yet the improvement seems to be isolated to respiratory outcomes and there is good evidence that epidural analgesia decreases respiratory complications (41).

SUMMARY

Regional analgesia is an integral component of a post-thoracotomy pain management protocol. Epidural analgesia can decrease morbidity and mortality following thoracotomy and this decrease seems to be most evident for patients at increased risk of postoperative respiratory complications. At present, the most convincing data suggest that this benefit is primarily with thoracic epidural infusions of opioids and local anesthetics. Clinically, the analgesia from a multimodal technique that incorporates continuous paravertebral blockade can approach that seen with epidural analgesia. It is not yet known if paravertebral analgesia can provide the same improvements in outcome that have been seen with epidural analgesia.

References

1. Nakahara K, Monden Y, Ohno K, Miyoshi S, Maeda H, Kawashima Y: A method for predicting postoperative lung function and its relation to postoperative complications in patients with lung cancer. Ann Thorac Surg 39:260–265, 1985
2. Nakahara K, Ohno K, Hashimoto J, Miyoshi S, Maeda H, Matsumura A, Mizuta T, Akashi A, Nakagawa K, Yasunaru Y: Prediction of postoperative respiratory failure in patients undergoing lung resection for cancer. Ann Thorac Surg 46:549–552, 1988
3. Cerfolio RJ, Allen MS, Trastek VF, Deschampcs C, Scanlon PD, Pairolero P: Lung resection in patients with compromised pulmonary function. Ann Thorac Surg 62:348–351, 1996
4. Licker M, de Perrot M, Hohn L, Tschopp J-M, Robert J, Frey J-G,

Schweizer A, Spiliopoulos A: Perioperative mortality and major cardio-pulmonary complications after lung surgery for non-small carcinoma. Eur J Cardio-thorac Surg 15:314–319, 1999

5. Ali J, Weisel RD, Layug AB, Kripke BJ, Hechtman HB: Consequences of postoperative alterations in respiratory mechanics. Am J Surg 128:376–82, 1974

6. Landreau RJ, Pigula F, Luketich JD: Acute and chronic morbidity differences between muscle-sparing and standard lateral thoracotomy: J Thorac Cardiovasc Surg 112:1346–1351, 1996

7. Shulman M, Sandler AN, Bradley JW, Brebner J: Postthoracotomy pain and pulmonary function following epidural and systemic morphine. Anesthesiology 61:569–575, 1984

8. Kavanagh BP, Katz J, Sandler AN: Pain control after thoracic surgery. A review of current techniques. Anesthesiology 81:737–759, 1994

9. Pavy T, Medley C, Murphy F: Effect of indomethacin on pain relief after thoracotomy. Br J Anaesth 65:624–627,1990

10. Dahl JB, Raeder JC: Non-opioid post-operative analgesia. Acta Anaesthesiol Scand 44: 1191–1203, 2000

11. Eide PK, Stubhaug A, Brevik H, Oye I: Ketamine relief from chronic pain through actions at the NMDA receptor. Pain 72:289–291, 1997

12. Dich-Nielson JO, Svendsen L, Berthelsen P: Intramuscular low dose Ketamine versus pethidine for postoperative pain treatment after thoracic surgery. Acta Anaesthesiol Scand 36:583–587, 1992

13. Chow TKF, Penberthy AJ, Goodchild CS: Ketamine as an adjunct to morphine in postthoracotomy analgesia. Anesth Analg 87:1372–1374, 1998

14. Moore DC, Bush WH, Scurlock JE: Intercostal nerve block: A roentgenographic anatomic study of technique and absorption in humans. Anesth Analg 59:815–825, 1980

15. Dryden CM, McMenemin I, Duthie DJ. Efficacy of continuous intercostal bupivacaine for pain relief after thoracotomy. Brit J Anaesth 70:508–510, 1993

16. Hardy PAJ: Anatomical variation in the position of the proximal intercostal nerve. Br J Anaesth 61:338–339, 1988

17. Crossley AWA, Hosie HE: Radiographic study of intercostal nerve blockade in healthy volunteers. Br J Anaesth 59:149–154, 1987

18. Fagiano G, Borasio P, Salamino A, Sodero A, Ricci C, Ardissone F: Risultat immediati e a distanza del crio-bloco dei nervi intercostali. Minerva Anestesiologica 51:39–43, 1985

19. Mueller LC, Salzer G, Ransmayer G: Intraoperative cryoanalgesia for post-thoracotomy pain relief. Ann Thorac Surg 18:15–18, 1989

20. Dajczman E, Gordon A, Kreisman H, Wolkove N: Long term post-thoracotomy pain. Chest 99:270–274, 1991

21. Gough JD, Williams AB, Vaughn RS: The control of post-thoracotomy pain. A comparative evaluation of thoracic epidural fentanyl infusions and cryoanalgesia. Anaesthesia 43: 780–783, 1988
22. Roviaro GC, Varoli F, Fascianella A, Mariani C, Ramella G, Ceccopieri AM, Pezzuoli G: Intrathoracic intercostal nerve block with phenol in open chest surgery. Chest 90:64–67, 1986
23. Symreng T, Gomez MN, Rossi N: Intrapleural bupivacaine v saline after thoracotomy—effects on pain and lung function—a double-blind study. J Cardiothorac Anesth 3:144–149, 1989
24. Brockmeier V, Moen H, Karlsson BR, Fjeld NB, Reiestad F, Steen PA: Interpleural or thoracic epidural analgesia for pain after thoracotomy. Acta Anaesthesiol Scand 38:317–321, 1993
25. Schnieder RF, Villamena PC, Harvey J, Surick BG, Surick IW, Beattie EJ: Lack of efficacy of intrapleural bupivacaine for postoperative analgesia following thoracotomy. Chest 103: 414–416, 1993
26. Bachmann-Mennenga B, Biscoping J, Kuhn DFM, Schurg R, Ryan B, Erkens U, Hemplemann G: Intercostal nerve block, interpleural analgesia, thoracic epidural block or systemic opioid for pain relief after thoracotomy? Eur J Cardiothorac Surg 7:12–18, 1993
27. Richardson J, Lonnqvist PA: Thoracic paravertebral block. Br J Anaesth 81:230–238, 1998
28. Berrisford RG, Sabanathan SS: Direct access to the paravertebral space at thoracotomy. Ann Thorac Surg 49:854, 1990
29. Watson DS, Panian S, Kendall V, Maher DP, Peters G: Pain control after thoracotomy: bupivacaine versus lidocaine in continuous extrapleural intercostal nerve blockade. Ann Thorac Surg 67:825–829, 1999
30. Karmakar MJ, Chung DC: Variability of a thoracic paravertebral block. Reg Anesth Pain Med 25:325–327, 2000
31. Cheema SPS, Isley D, Richardson J, Sabanathan S: A thermographic study of paravertebral analgesia. Anaesthesia 50:116–121, 1995
32. Perttunen K, Nilsson E, Heinonen J, Hirvisalo E-L, Salo JA, Kalso E: Extradural, paravertebral and intercostal nerve blocks for post-thoracotomy pain. Br J Anaesth 75:541–547, 1995
33. Shah R, Sabanathan S, Richardson J, Mearns A, Bembridge J : Continuous paravertebral block for post thoracotomy analgesia in children. J Cardiovasc Surg 38:543–6, 1997
34. Dauphin A, Gupta RN, Young JE, Morton WD: Serum bupivacaine concentrations during continuous extrapleural infusion. Can J Anaesth 44:367–70, 1997
35. Soni AK, Conacher I, Waller DA, Hilton CJ: Video-assisted thoracoscopic placement of paravertebral catheters. Br J Anaesth 72:462–464, 1994

36. Benedetti F, Amazanio M, Casadio C: Control of postoperative pain by transcutaneous electrical nerve stimulation after thoracic operations. Ann Thorac Surg 63:773–776, 1997
37. Stubbing JF, Jellicoe JA: Transcutaneuous electrical nerve stimulation after thoracotomy. Anaesthesia 43:296–298, 1988
38. Warfield CA, Stein JM, Frank HA: The effect of transcutaneous electrical nerve stimulation on pain after thoracotomy. Ann Thorac Surg 39:462–465, 1985
39. Corning JL: Spinal anesthesia and local medications of the cord. NY Med J Oct. 31, 42:483, 1885.
40. Cohen E, Neustein SM: Intrathecal morphine during thoracotomy: J Cardiothorac Anesth 7:154–163, 1993
41. Ballantyne JC, Carr DB, deFerranti S: The comparative effects of postoperative analgesic therapies on pulmonary outcome: Cumulative meta-analysis of randomized, controlled trials. Anesth Analg 86:598–612, 1998
42. Slinger P, Shennib H, Wilson S: Postthoracotomy pulmonary function: a comparison of epidural versus intravenous meperidine infusions. J Cardiothorac Vasc Anesth 9:128–134, 1995
43. Cook TM, Riley RH: Analgesia following thoracotomy: A survey of Australian practice. Anaesth Intens Care 25:520–524, 1997
44. Rodgers A, Walker N, Schug S, McKee A, Kehlet H, van Zundert A, Sage D, Futter M, Saville G, Clark T, MacMahon S: Reduction of postoperative mortality and morbidity with epidural or spinal anesthesia: results from an overview of randomized trials. Br Med J 321:1–12, 2000
45. Mourisse J, Hasenbros M, Gielen M: Epidural bupivacaine, sufentanil or the combination for post-thoracotomy pain. Acta Anaesthesiol Scan 36:70–74, 1992
46. Wiebalck A, Brodner G, Van Aken H: The effects of adding sufentanil to bupivacaine for post-operative patient contraolled analgesia. Anesth Analg 85:124–129, 1997
47. George KA, Wright PMC, Chrisakuta A: Continuous thoracic epidural for post-thoracotomy pain relief: with or without bupivacaine. Anaesthesia 46:732–736, 1991
48. Hansdottir V, Wostenborghs R, Nordberg G: The pharmocokinetics of continuous epidural sufentanil and bupivacaine infusions after thoracotomy. Anesth Analg 83:394–406, 1996
49. Etches RC, Sander AN, Daly MD: Respiratory depression and spinal opioids. Can J Anaesth 36:165–185, 1989
50. Shuman RL, Peters RM: Epidural anesthesia following thoracotomy in patients with chronic obstructive airway disease. J Thorac Cardiovasc Surg 71:82–88, 1976
51. Ready LB, Loper KA, Nessly M, Wild L: Postoperative epidural

morphine is safe on surgical wards. Anesthesiology 75:452–456, 1991

52. Moniche S, Hjortso N-C, Blemmer T: Blood pressure and heart rate during orthostatic stress and walking with continuous postoperative epidural bupivacaine/morphine. Acta Anaesthesiol Scand 37:65–69, 1993

53. Giebler RM, Scherer RU, Peters J: Incidence of neurologic complications related to thoracic epidural catheterization. Anesthesiology 86:55–63, 1997

54. Slinger PD: Pro: every postthoracotomy patient deserves thoracic epidural analgesia. J Cardiothorac Vasc Anesth 13:350–354, 1999

55. Tejwani GA, Rattan AK , McDonald JS: Role of spinal opioid receptors in the antinociceptive interactions between intrathecal morphine and bupivacaine. Anesth Analg. 84:726–734, 1992

56. Dales RE, Dionne G, Leech JA: Preoperative prediction of pulmonary complications following thoracic surgery. Chest 104:155–159, 1993.

57. Pansard JL, Mankikian B, Bertrand M, Kieffer E, Clergue F, Viars P: Effects of thoracic extradural block on diaphragmatic electrical activity and contractility after upper abdominal surgery. Anesthesiology 78:63–71, 1993

58. Polaner DM, Kimball WR, Fratacci M-D: Improvement of diaphragmatic function by a thoracic epidural block after upper abdominal surgery. Anesthesiology 79:808–816, 1993

59. Fratacci M-D, Kimball WR, Wain JC: Diaphragmatic shortening after thoracic surgery in humans. Anesthesiology 79:654–665, 1993

60. Warner DO, Warner MA, Ritman EL: Human chest wall function during epidural anesthesia. Anesthesiology 85:761–773, 1996

61. Wahba WM, Craig DB, Don HF, Becklake MR: The cardiorespiratory effects of thoracic epidural analgesia. Can Anaesth Soc J 19:8–19, 1972

62. Craig DB. Postoperative recovery of pulmonary function. Anesth Analg 60:46–52,1981

63. Gruber EM, Tschernko EM, Kritzinger M,Deviatko E, Wisser W, Zurakowski D, Haider W: The effects of thoracic epidural analgesia with bupivacaine 0.25% on ventilatory mechanics in patients with severe chronic obstructive pulmonary disease. Anesth Analg 92:1015–1019, 2001

64. Von Knorring J, Lepantalo J, Lindgren L, Lindfors O: Cardiac arrhythmias and myocardial ischemia after thoracotomy for lung cancer. Ann Thorac Surg 53:642–547, 1992

65. Amar D, Burt M, Reinsel RA, Leung DHY: Relationship of early post-operative dysrhythmias and long-term outcome after rescection of non-small cell lung cancer. Chest 110:437–439, 1996

66. Staats PS, Panchal SJ: Thoracic epidural analgesia for treatment of angina. J Cardiothorac Vasc Anesth 11:105–108, 1997

67. Backlund M, Laasonen L, Leptantalo: Effect of oxygen on pulmonary hemodynamics and incidence of atrial fibrillation after noncardiac thoracic surgery. J Cardiothorac Vasc Anesth 12:422–428, 1998

68. Lindgren L, Lepantalo M, Von Knorring J: Effect of verapamil on right ventricular pressure and atrial tachyarrhythmias after thoracotomy. Br J Anaesth 66:205–211, 1991

69. Meissner A, Rolf N, Van Aken H: Thoracic epidural anesthesia and patients with heart disease: benefits, risks and controversies. Anesth Analg 85:517–528, 1997

70. Saada M, Catoire P, Bonnet F: Effect of thoracic epidural anesthesia combined with general anesthesia on segmental wall motion assessed by transesophageal echocardiography. Anesth Analg 75:329–335, 1991

71. Saada M, Duval A-M, Bonnet F: Abnormalities in myocardial wall motion during lumbar epidural anesthesia. Anesth Analg 71:26–33, 1989

72. Armstrong P: Thoracic epidural anaesthesia and primary pulmonary hypertension. Anaesthesia 47:496–499, 1992

73. Visser WA, liem TH, van Egmond J, Gielen MJM: Extension of sensory blockade after thoracic epidural administration ot a test dose of lidocaine at three different levels. Anesth Analg 86:332–335, 1998

74. Hendriks GWH, Hasenbos MAWM, Gielen MJM, Egmond JV, Barentsz JO: Evaluation of thoracic epidural catheter position and migration using radio-opaque catheters. Anaesthesia 52:457–459, 1997

75. Cousins M: Comparative pharmacokinetics of spinal opioids in humans. Anesthesiology 67:875–876,1987

76. Niemi G, Breivik H: Adrenaline markedly improves thoracic epidural analgesia produced by a low dose infusion of bupivacaine, fentanyl and adrenaline after major surgery. Acta Anaesthesiol Scand 42: 897–909, 1998

77. Romer HC, Russell GN: A survey of the practice of thoracic epidural analgesia in the United Kingdom. Anaesthesia 53: 1016–1022, 1998

78. Horlocker TT, Caplan RA: Should regional blockade be performed on anesthetized patients? ASA Newsletter 65(4): 5–7, 2001

79. de Leon-Casasola OA, Yarussi A: Physiopathology of opioid tolerance and clinical approach to the opioid tolerant patient. Curr Rev Pain 4:203–205, 2000

80. de Leon-Casasola OA, Lema MJ: Epidural bupivicaine/sufentanil

therapy for postoperative pain control in patients tolerant to opioid and unresponsive to epidural bupivicaine/morphine. Anesthesiology 80:303–309, 1994.

81. Schmid R, Sandler AN, Katz J: Use and efficacy of low dose ketamine in the management of acute postoperative pain. Pain 82:111–115, 1999

82. Mukaida T, Andou A, Date H, Aoe M, Shimizu N: Thoracoscopic operation for secondary pneumothorax under local and epidural anesthesia. Ann Thorac Surg 65:924–926, 1998

83. Williams A, Kay J: Thoracic epidural anesthesia for thoracoscopy, rib resection, and thoracotomy in a patient with bronchopleural fistula postpneumonectomy. Anesthesiology 92:1482–1484, 2000

84. Kahn L, Baxter F, Dauphin A, Goldschmidt C, Jackson PA, McChesney J, Miller JD, Young JEM: A comparison of thoracic and lumbar epidurals techniques for post-thoracoabdominal esophagectomy analgesia. Can J Anesth 46:415–422, 1999

Terese T. Horlocker, M.D.

Regional Anesthesia and Anticoagulation: Are the Benefits Worth the Risks?

8

INTRODUCTION

Spinal hematoma is a rare and potentially catastrophic complication of spinal or epidural anesthesia. The first spinal anesthetic was administered by Bier in 1898. Ten years later, the first spinal hematoma following neuraxial blockade was recorded. Sollier (1) reported permanent paralysis in a 36-year-old male after unsuccessful spinal anesthesia for excision of a pilonidal cyst. Ten days later, the patient complained of paresthesias and weakness of his lower extremities. Lumbar radiograph demonstrated spina bifida occulta, while dilated spinal veins consistent with a vascular tumor were noted during decompressive laminectomy. Neurologic recovery was poor. Although there was no evidence for a pre-existing coagulopathy, the spina bifida occulta and vascular malformation were regarded as risk factors contributing to the development of spinal hematoma.

Patients with pre-existing coagulopathies have historically been considered at increased risk for hemorrhagic complications following neuraxial blockade. In 1953, the first spinal hematoma in a patient with altered hemostasis was noted by Bonica (2). The patient complained of signs consistent with cauda equina syndrome 4 days after bloody spinal puncture. Exploratory laminectomy revealed extensive clots within the subarachnoid space, which were compressing the conus medullaris. Hemostasis was difficult due to continued intrathecal bleeding. The wound was packed, exacerbating neurologic ischemia, and the patient sustained irreversible neurologic injury.

Regional Anesthesia for Cardiothoracic Surgery, edited by Mark Chaney,
Lippincott Williams & Wilkins, Baltimore © 2002.

The clinical introduction of heparin in 1937, and coumarin derivatives in 1941, heralded new concerns regarding the regional anesthetic management of perioperatively anticoagulated patients . However, the relative rarity of spinal hematoma, as well as the publication of several large studies reported over the last two decades (3–7), increased the clinician's confidence in management of the anticoagulated patient undergoing neuraxial blockade. A new challenge occurred with the release of low molecular weight heparin (LMWH) for general use in the United States in May 1993. The pharmacologic differences between LMWH and standard heparin were underestimated; over 40 spinal hematomas were reported through the MedWatch system over a 5-year period. This experience contrasted dramatically with that of European clinicians who had reported only 13 spinal hematomas in patients receiving LMWH despite a decade of extensive clinical use (6). The marked increase in the frequency of spinal hematoma in patients anticoagulated with LMWH prompted a re-evaluation of the relative risks and benefits of neuraxial blockade in the anticoagulated patient.

This review will discuss the incidence and risk factors for spinal hematoma, the beneficial effects of neuraxial anesthesia and analgesia, and the perioperative indications for thromboprophylaxis. An understanding of the pharmacologic properties of anticoagulants and antiplatelet medications, and the clinical studies and case reports involving patients undergoing central neural blockade while receiving these medications is paramount in reducing the risk of spinal hematoma in patients undergoing neuraxial blockade. Recommendations for patient management reported in this review follow the consensus statements on Neuraxial Anesthesia and Anticoagulation published by the American Society of Regional Anesthesia (8–12).

BENEFICIAL EFFECTS OF NEURAXIAL ANESTHESIA AND ANALGESIA

Spinal and epidural anesthesia/analgesia provide several advantages over systemic opioids, including superior analgesia, reduced blood loss and need for transfusion, and decreased incidence of thromboembolic complications (13). It is current medical practice that patients hospitalized for major surgery often receive an anticoagulant and/or antiplatelet medication perioperatively to prevent venous thrombosis and pulmonary embolism, although the pharmacologic agent, degree of anticoagulation desired, and duration of therapy remain controversial (Table 9–1). In the United States, oral anticoagulants and LMWH are most often utilized in patients undergoing major orthopedic surgery, while low-dose (unfractionated) heparin or aspirin may be used in pa-

TABLE 8–1.   Pharmacological Venous Thromboembolism Prophylaxis and Treatment Regimens, and Treatment Regimens for Acute Coronary Syndromes

Indication and Modality	Regimen
Venous thromboembolism prophylaxis	
Total Hip or Knee Replacement	
Adjusted-dose unfractionated heparin	3,500 U SC Q8 hours, started 2 hours before surgery; after surgery, the dose is adjusted to maintain the aPTT within the upper normal range
Low molecular weight heparin	
Ardeparin sodium (Normiflo®)	50 IU/kg SC BID, started 12–24 hours after surgery
Dalteparin sodium (Fragmin®)	5000 IU SC QD, started 12 hours before surgery, or 2500 IU SC given 7 hours after surgery, then 5000 IU SC daily
Danaparoid sodium (Orgaran®)	750 U SC BID, started 2 hours before surgery
Enoxaparin sodium (Lovenox®)	30 mg SC BID, started 12–24 hours after surgery, or 40 mg SC QD, started 10–12 hours before surgery
Tinzaparin sodium (Innohep®)	75 IU/kg SC QD, started 10–12 hours before surgery
Warfarin sodium	5 mg PO, started the night before or immediately after surgery and adjusted to prolong the INR=2.0–3.0
General Surgery	
Unfractionated heparin	5,000 U SC Q8–12 hours, started 2 hours before surgery
Low molecular weight heparin	
Dalteparin sodium	2500 IU SC QD, started 1–2 hours before surgery
Enoxaparin sodium	40 mg SC QD, started 2 hours before surgery
Venous thromboembolism therapy	
Enoxaparin sodium (Lovenox®)	1 mg/kg SC Q12 hours (outpatient deep vein thrombosis)
	1 mg/kg SC Q12 hours, or 1.5 mg/kg SC QD (inpatient treatment of deep vein thrombosis or pulmonary embolism)
Nadroparin calcium (Fraxiparine®)	200 U/kg SC Q 12 hours
Tinzaparin (Innohep®)	175 U/kg SC daily
Acute coronary syndromes	
Enoxaparin sodium (Lovenox®)	1 mg/kg SC Q12 hours. Concurrent aspirin therapy recommended.
Dalteparin sodium (Fragmin®)	120 U/kg Q12 hours. Concurrent aspirin therapy recommended.

tients undergoing thoracoabdominal surgery or in elderly or debilitated patients where increased risk of hemorrhage is present. Patients receiving perioperative thromboprophylaxis are often not considered candidates for spinal or epidural anesthesia/analgesia because of a theoretically greater risk of spinal hematoma. The decision to perform neuraxial blockade on these patients must be made on an individual basis, weighing the risk of spinal hematoma from needle or catheter placement against the theoretical benefits gained.

The improved perioperative outcome associated with neuraxial anesthesia and analgesia is related to superior analgesia and an attenuation of the surgical stress response. Surgical stress activates the sympathetic nervous system, and is believed to be an indirect cause of adverse cardiac, pulmonary, gastrointestinal, and immune outcomes. For example, cardiac morbidity may be increased through the release of neuroendocrine hormones (epinephrine, norepinephrine, cortisol, renin) with resultant increase in oxygen demand or decrease in oxygen supply. The stress response potentiates the development of a hypercoagulable state that predisposes to thromboembolic events. Finally, stress response mediators are potent inhibitors of the immune system, and may contribute to immunosuppression and infection. It is important to note that the benefits of neuraxial anesthesia and analgesia vary according to patient population and surgical procedure. The differences in outcome are most impressive in high-risk populations undergoing major surgery (13).

Cardiac and Lower Extremity Revascularization Procedures

The patient undergoing cardiovascular surgery presents a regional anesthetic management dilemma to the anesthesiologist. Multiple studies have demonstrated the beneficial effects on coagulation status and perioperative outcome associated with neuraxial anesthesia and analgesia in patients undergoing major vascular surgery. However, these patients frequently receive antiplatelet medications, anticoagulants, and/or thrombolytic drugs perioperatively. As a result, hemostasis may not be normal until several days after surgery. Removal of an indwelling neuraxial catheter requires a partial or complete resolution of the anticoagulant effects. The potential for bleeding into the spinal canal must be balanced with lower extremity graft occlusion. Appropriate timing of catheter removal requires communication and compromise among the entire patient care team.

Major vascular surgery is associated with a hypercoagulable state that persists into the postoperative period. All components of the coagulation cascade are affected, including increased concentrations of coagulation factors, enhanced platelet activity, and impaired fibrinolysis. Epidural anesthesia and analgesia (with a local anesthetic-containing solution) attenuates the increases in postoperative coagulability and improves clinical outcome, especially among high-risk patient populations. Tuman et al.. (14) evaluated the effect of anesthetic technique on outcome in patients undergoing lower extremity revascularization. Patients were randomized to receive general anesthesia combined with epidural anesthesia and analgesia or general anesthesia combined with on-demand opioid analgesia. The patients receiving epidural anesthesia and analgesia had a lower incidence of thrombotic events (peripheral arterial graft, coronary artery, or deep venous thrombosis). In addition, the rates of cardiovascular, infectious, and overall complications, as well as the duration of stay in the intensive care unit, were also lower among these patients. These results have been duplicated in subsequent studies. However, as previously mentioned the differences in outcome were most marked in patients with significant pre-existing medical conditions undergoing suprainguinal (thoracic or abdominal aorta) vascular procedures.

The potential benefits of intrathecal and epidural anesthesia and analgesia for cardiac revascularization surgery remain undefined. Although the profound analgesia, attenuation of the stress response, and thoracic cardiac sympathectomy theoretically may be beneficial, there are few prospective randomized, placebo-controlled studies evaluating neuraxial block in patients undergoing cardiac surgery, and none uses clinical outcome as a primary endpoint (15). In a review summarizing the risks and benefits associated with intrathecal or epidural anesthesia and analgesia in patients undergoing cardiac surgery, the authors concluded that the effect of neuraxial block on outcome cannot be definitively determined given the current available data, and urged that additional studies be performed to determine the impact of neuraxial block on morbidity and mortality in cardiac surgical patients.

INCIDENCE AND RISK FACTORS FOR SPINAL HEMATOMA

The actual incidence of neurologic dysfunction resulting from hemorrhagic complications associated with central neural blockade is unknown; however, the incidence cited in the literature is estimated to be less than 1 in 150,000 epidural and less than 1 in 220,000 spinal anesthetics (16). Hemorrhage into the spinal canal most commonly occurs in the epidural space because of the prominent epidural venous plexus.

Although hemorrhagic complications can occur after virtually all regional anesthetic techniques, bleeding into the spinal canal is perhaps the most serious hemorrhagic complication associated with regional anesthesia because the spinal canal is a concealed and nonexpandable space. Spinal cord compression from spinal hematoma may result in neurologic ischemia and paraplegia. Spinal hematoma may occur due to vascular trauma from needle or catheter placement into the subarachnoid or epidural space. However, it may also occur in association with neoplastic disease or pre-existing vascular abnormalities. Of special interest to the anesthesiologist are those spinal hematomas that have occurred spontaneously with or without the presence of antiplatelet or anticoagulation therapy. Over 100 spontaneous epidural hematomas have been reported, 25% of which are associated with anticoagulation therapy (17).

In a review of the literature between 1906 and 1994, Vandermeulen et al. (18) reported 61 cases of spinal hematoma associated with epidural or spinal anesthesia. In 42 of the 61 patients (68%), the spinal hematomas associated with central neural blockade occurred in patients with evidence of hemostatic abnormality. Twenty-five of the patients had received intravenous or subcutaneous heparin, while an additional 5 patients were presumably administered heparin, as they were undergoing a vascular surgical procedure. In addition, 12 patients had evidence of coagulopathy or thrombocytopenia or were treated with antiplatelet medications (aspirin, indomethacin, ticlopidine), oral anticoagulants (phenprocoumone), thrombolytics (urokinase), or dextran 70 immediately before or after the spinal or epidural anesthetic. Needle and catheter placement was reported to be difficult in 15 (25%), or bloody in 15 (25%) patients. Thus, in 53 of the 61 cases (87%), either a clotting abnormality or needle placement difficulty was present.

Regional technique was also noted. A spinal anesthetic was performed in 15 patients. The remaining 46 patients received an epidural anesthetic, including 32 patients with an in-dwelling catheter. In 15 of these 32 patients, the spinal hematoma occurred immediately after the removal of the epidural catheter. (Nine of these catheters were removed during therapeutic levels of heparinization). These results suggest that catheter removal is not entirely atraumatic, and the patient's coagulation status at the time of catheter removal is perhaps as critical as that at the time of catheter placement.

Neurologic compromise presented as progression of sensory or motor block or bowel/bladder dysfunction, not severe radicular back pain. Importantly, although only 38% of patients had partial or good neurologic recovery, spinal cord ischemia tended to be reversible in patients who underwent laminectomy within 8 hours of onset of neurologic dysfunction (Table 9–2).

TABLE 8–2.   Neurologic Outcome in Patients with Spinal
Hematoma Following Neuraxial Blockade*

Interval Between Onset of Paraplegia and Surgery	Good N=15	Partial N=11	Poor N=29
Less than 8 hours (N=13)	6	4	3
Between 8 and 24 hours (N=7)	1	2	4
Greater than 24 hours (N=12)	2	0	10
No surgical intervention (N=13)	4	1	8
Unknown (N=10)	2	4	4

*Neurologic outcome was reported for 55 of 61 cases of spinal hematoma following neuraxial blockade
  Adapted from Vandermeulen EP, Van Aken H, Vermylen J: Anticoagulants and spinal-epidural anesthesia. Anesth Analg 79:1165–1177, 1994. With permission.

Intravenous Heparin

Heparin is a complex polysaccharide that exerts its anticoagulant effect by accelerating the inhibition of activated coagulation factors by antithrombin III. Activated clotting factors that are inhibited by antithrombin III include factors XIIa, XIa, Xa, and IXa and thrombin. Heparin also potentiates the action of activated factor X inhibitors (anti-Xa effect). The key position of factor X in the coagulation cascade enables it to generate thrombin through the intrinsic or extrinsic pathway. Therefore, inhibitors of this enzyme's activation will prevent thrombin formation. Five minutes after intravenous injection of 10,000 units of heparin, the coagulation time is prolonged 2 to 4 times the control level. Heparin has a half-life in circulating blood of 1 1/2 to 2 hours. Patients with acute thromboembolic disease may clear heparin even more rapidly. Within 4 to 6 hours of the administration of a therapeutic dose of heparin, its effect has ceased. Intravenously administered heparin can be promptly neutralized by protamine.

In perhaps the most important study evaluating the safety of systemic heparinization and central neural blockade, Rao and El-Etr (5) reported on 3,164 patients who had continuous epidural anesthesia and 847 patients who had continuous spinal anesthesia for lower extremity vascular procedures. Patients with a history of pre-existing coagulation abnormalities, thrombocytopenia, or preoperative anticoagulation therapy were excluded. All catheters were placed through a 17-gauge Tuohy needle. In 4 patients, following insertion of the needle into the epidural space, blood was freely aspirated. The needle was withdrawn and the patients were given general anesthesia the following day. Heparin was administered 50 to 60 minutes after catheter placement to maintain the activated clotting time (ACT) twice the baseline value. The heparin dose was repeated every 6 hours following measurement of the ACT throughout the period of anticoagulation therapy. The catheters were removed the following day 1hour prior to administration of the maintenance dose of heparin. No patient developed signs or symptoms of epidural or subarachnoid hematoma, including the 4 patients who had traumatic needle placement and subsequently received general anesthesia. In summary, while the patients in this study safely underwent placement of in-dwelling epidural or spinal catheters followed by systemic heparinization, the heparin activity was closely monitored and the in-dwelling catheters were removed at a time when circulating heparin levels were relatively low. There were also no neurologic sequelae reported by Baron et al. (19) in 912 vascular surgical patients who received continuous epidural anesthesia and underwent transient intraoperative anticoagulation with heparin (aPTT>100 seconds). The catheters were removed immediately after surgery.

Mathews and Abrams (20) reported no neurologic complications in 40 cardiac surgical patients who received intrathecal morphine through 20- to 25-gauge needles 50 minutes prior to cardiopulmonary bypass (and complete anticoagulation with heparin). Subsequent authors have demonstrated similar good outcomes with both single and continuous techniques in patients undergoing cardiopulmonary bypass. In a review of the literature in 1997, Chaney (15) was able to document that intrathecal anesthesia and/or analgesia had been administered to 771 patients prior to cardiopulmonary bypass. An additional 417 patients received continuous epidural techniques. In-dwelling catheters were placed the night before surgery, immediately preoperatively or postoperatively. Surgery was often canceled or delayed if blood was present during needle or catheter placement. It is important to note that there were no reported cases of spinal hematoma among these patients (15) or within the American Society of Anesthesiologist Closed Claims Project (21). In a survey of the membership of the Society of Cardiovascular Anesthesiologists, 7.6% of responders use spinal techniques and 7.0% reported they use epidural techniques for cardiac surgery (22). Interestingly, the majority of anesthesiologists would proceed with surgery if frank blood was noted in the spinal or epidural needle. Once again, there were no reported hematomas or neurologic complications among the respondents.

Although the previous studies suggest that central neural blockade (in the presence of an in-dwelling catheter) followed by heparinization can be safely conducted, Ruff and Dougherty (23) reported documented spinal hematomas in 7 of 342 patients (2%) who underwent a diagnostic lumbar puncture with a 20-gauge needle. The patients presented with signs of cerebral ischemia, and after subarachnoid hemorrhage was ruled out, they were subsequently anticoagulated with intravenous heparin. The amount of heparin used and coagulation studies were not reported. Five patients developed paraparesis. There were also 18 patients with severe or radicular back pain lasting more than 48 hours. Seven of these patients subsequently died of unrelated causes, and at autopsy, 1 patient had findings of chronic epidural hematoma while another showed an organized subdural hematoma. The authors identified traumatic needle placement, initiation of anticoagulation within 1 hour of lumbar puncture or concomitant aspirin therapy as being risk factors in the development of spinal hematoma in anticoagulated patients.

The conflicting results of these studies and the rarity of this complication make it difficult to assess the relative risk and contributing variables of spinal hematoma associated with continuous catheter techniques of central neural blockade in anticoagulated patients. However, possible factors contributing to increased risk in these patients appear to be pre-existing coagulopathy or thrombocytopenia, concomitant aspirin therapy, traumatic or difficult needle placement, heparinization within 1 hour of spinal or epidural puncture, and absence of monitoring the anticoagulant activity (5, 20, 23).

Subcutaneous Heparin

The therapeutic basis of low-dose subcutaneous heparin (5000 units every 8–12 hours) is based on heparin-mediated inhibition of activated factor X. Inhibition of small amounts of activated factor X prevents amplification of the coagulation cascade. Smaller doses of heparin are therefore required when administered as prophylaxis rather than as treatment for thromboembolic disease. Following intramuscular or subcutaneous injection of 5000 units of heparin, maximum anticoagulation effect is observed in 40 to 50 minutes and usually returns to baseline within 4 to 6 hours. The activated partial thromboplastin time (aPTT) may remain in the normal range and often is not monitored. However, wide variation in individual patient response to subcutaneous heparin has been reported (24). This wide variation in response to subcutaneous low-dose heparin makes it difficult to formulate a generalized recommendation regarding central neural blockade in these patients. Lowson and Goodchild (25) and Allemann et al . (26) reported no cases of spinal hematoma in a combined total of 204 epidural and 119 spinal anesthetics performed on patients who had received 5000 U of unfractionated heparin subcutaneously 2 hours prior to needle placement. A review of the literature by Schwander and Bachmann (7) in 1991 noted no spinal hematomas in over 5000 patients who received varying doses of subcutaneous heparin in combination with spinal or epidural anesthesia. Spinal hematoma in patients who undergo major conduction blocks while receiving low-dose heparin are extremely rare; there are only three reported cases in the literature, two of which involved a continuous epidural anesthetic technique (27–29).

Regional Anesthetic Management of the Patient Receiving Standard Heparin

The safety of neuraxial techniques in combination with intraoperative heparinization is well documented, providing no other coagulopathies are present. The concurrent use of medications that affect other components of the clotting mechanisms may increase the risk of bleeding complications for patients receiving standard heparin. These medications include antiplatelet medications, LMWH, and oral anticoagulants (8).

Intravenous heparin administration should be delayed for 1 hour after needle placement. In-dwelling catheters should be removed 1 hour before a subsequent heparin administration or 2 to 4 hours after the last heparin dose. Evaluation of the coagulation status may be appropriate prior to catheter removal in patients who have demonstrated enhanced response or are on higher doses of heparin. Although the occurrence of a bloody or difficult needle placement may increase risk, there are no data to support mandatory cancellation of a case should this occur. If the decision is made to proceed, full discussion with the surgeon and careful postoperative monitoring are warranted (8).

Prolonged therapeutic anticoagulation appears to increase risk of spinal hematoma formation, especially if combined with other anticoagulants or thrombolytics. Therefore, neuraxial blocks should be avoided in this clinical setting. If systematic anticoagulation therapy is begun with an epidural catheter in place, it is recommended to delay catheter removal for 2 to 4 hours following heparin discontinuation and after evaluation of coagulation status (8).

There is no contraindication to use of neuraxial techniques during subcutaneous standard heparin. The risk of neuraxial bleeding may be reduced by delay of the heparin injection until after the block, and may be increased in debilitated patients or after prolonged therapy (8).

Low Molecular Weight Heparin

Unfractionated heparin is a heterogenous mixture of polysaccharide chains that can be separated into fragments of various molecular weights. Since each LMWH fractionation contains heparins of different molecular weights, each must be evaluated as a specific pharmacological substance. LMWH exhibits a dose-dependent antithrombotic effect that is most accurately assessed by measuring the anti-Xa activity level.

However, the anti-Xa level is not predictive of hemorrhagic complications and is typically not monitored. The advantages of LMWH over unfractionated heparin include a higher and more predictable bioavailability after subcutaneous administration, a longer biologic half-life that makes one injection per day sufficient for some patient populations, and a smaller impact on platelet function (30). Peak anti-Xa activity occurs 3 to 4 hours after a subcutaneous LMWH injection, and 12-hour anti-Xa levels are approximately 50% of peak levels. The plasma half-life of LMWH is approximately 2 to 4 times longer than that of unfractionated heparin and increases in patients with renal failure (30).

LMWH has been approved for thromboprophylaxis following knee or hip arthroplasty, abdominal surgery, and treatment of acute thromboembolism or non-q-wave myocardial infarction (Table 9–1). Extensive clinical testing and utilization of LMWH in Europe over the last 10 years suggests that there is not an increased risk of spinal hematoma in patients undergoing neuraxial anesthesia while receiving LMWH thromboprophylaxis perioperatively (6, 18). However, in the 5 years since the release of LMWH for general use in the United States in May 1993, over 40 cases of spinal hematoma associated with neuraxial anesthesia administered in the presence of perioperative LMWH prophylaxis have been reported to the manufacturer (9). Many of these events occurred when LMWH was administered intraoperatively or early postoperatively to patients undergoing continuous epidural anesthesia and analgesia. Concomitant antiplatelet therapy was present in several cases. The apparent difference in incidence in Europe compared to the United States may be a result of a difference in dose and dosage schedule. For example, in Europe the recommended dose of enoxaparin is 40 mg once daily, rather than 30 mg every 12 hours. However, timing of catheter removal may also have an impact. Although the actual frequency of spinal hematoma in patients receiving enoxaparin while undergoing spinal or epidural anesthesia is difficult to determine, the incidence has been estimated to be 1 in 3,100 continuous epidural anesthetics and 1 in 41,000 spinal anesthetics (31). Continued evaluation of the safety of spinal or epidural anesthesia in a patient receiving LMWH prophylaxis is required. Indeed, it appears that the clinician should proceed cautiously with regional anesthesia in the patient receiving LMWH.

Regional Anesthetic Management of the Patient Receiving LMWH

Anesthesiologists in the United States can draw upon the European experience to develop their own practice guidelines for the management of patients undergoing spinal and epidural blocks while receiving perioperative LMWH. Monitoring of the anti-Xa level is not recommended.

The anti-Xa level is not predictive of the risk of bleeding, and is therefore not helpful in the management of patients undergoing neuraxial blocks (9).

Antiplatelet or oral anticoagulant medications administered in combination with LMWH may increase the risk of spinal hematoma. Concomitant administration of medications affecting hemostasis, such as antiplatelet drugs, standard heparin, or dextran represents an additional risk of hemorrhagic complications perioperatively, including spinal hematoma. Education of the entire patient care team is necessary to avoid potentiation of the anticoagulant effects (9).

Patients on preoperative LMWH can be assumed to have altered coagulation at the time of needle placement. A single-dose spinal anesthetic may be the safest neuraxial technique in patients receiving preoperative LMWH. In these patients, needle placement should occur at least 10 to 12 hours after the LMWH dose. This is consistent with European regimens, where the first dose is administered 12 hours preoperatively. Patients receiving higher "treatment" doses of LMWH (e.g., enoxaparin 1 mg/kg twice daily) will require longer delays (24 hours). Neuraxial techniques should be avoided in patients administered a dose of LMWH 2 hours preoperatively (general surgery patients), since needle placement occurs during peak anticoagulant activity (9).

Patients with postoperative initiation of LMWH thromboprophylaxis may safely undergo single-dose and continuous catheter techniques. The first dose of LMWH should be administered no earlier than 24 hours postoperatively. In addition, it is recommended that indwelling catheters be removed prior to initiation of LMWH thromboprophylaxis. If a continuous technique is selected, the epidural catheter may be left in-dwelling overnight and removed the following day, with the first dose of LMWH administered 2 hours after catheter removal (9).

The decision to implement LMWH thromboprophylaxis in the presence of an in-dwelling catheter must be made with care. Extreme vigilance of the patient's neurologic status is warranted. An opioid or dilute local anesthetic solution is recommended in these patients in order to allow frequent monitoring of neurologic function. If epidural analgesia is anticipated to continue for more than 24 hours, LMWH administration may be delayed, or an alternate method of thromboprophylaxis may be selected (e.g., external pneumatic compression), based on the risk profile for the individual patient. These decisions should be made preoperatively to allow optimal management of both postoperative analgesia and thromboprophylaxis (9).

For any LMWH prophylaxis regimen, timing of catheter removal is of paramount importance. Catheter removal should be delayed for at least 10 to 12 hours after a dose of LMWH. A true normalization of the patient's coagulation status could be achieved if the evening dose of

LMWH was not given and the catheter was removed the following morning (24 hours after the last dose). Again, subsequent dosing should not occur for at least 2 hours after catheter removal (9).

Oral Anticoagulants

Oral anticoagulants, including warfarin, exert their anticoagulant effect indirectly by interfering with the synthesis of the vitamin K-dependent clotting factors (VII, IX, X, and thrombin). The effects of warfarin are not apparent until a significant amount of biologically inactive factors are synthesized. Since factor VII has a relatively short half-life (6–8 hours), the prothrombin time (PT) may be prolonged into the therapeutic range (1.5–2 times normal) in 24 to 36 hours. Since factor VII participates only in the extrinsic pathway, adequate anticoagulation is not achieved until the levels of biologically active factors II and X are sufficiently depressed, which, because of their longer half-lives, requires 4 to 6 days. With initial high loading doses of warfarin (15–30 mg) for the first 2 to 3 days of therapy, the desired anticoagulant effect is achieved within 48 to 72 hours. However, a higher frequency of bleeding complications has also been associated with use of a warfarin loading dose. Similarly, the anticoagulant effects persist for 4 to 6 days after termination of therapy while new biologically active vitamin K factors are synthesized; adequate levels of factors II, IX, and X (as well as factor VII) are present only when the international normalized ratio has normalized (10). In an emergent situation, the anticoagulant effects can be reversed by transfusing fresh frozen plasma and vitamin K injections.

Few data exist regarding the risk of spinal hematoma in patients with in-dwelling spinal or epidural catheters who are subsequently anticoagulated with warfarin. Odoom and Sih (4) performed 1,000 continuous lumbar epidural anesthetics in 950 patients undergoing vascular procedures who were receiving oral anticoagulants preoperatively. The thrombotest (a test measuring factor IX activity) was decreased and the aPTT was prolonged in all patients prior to needle placement. A modest heparin infusion was administered intraoperatively. Epidural catheters remained in place for 48 hours postoperatively; the coagulation status at time of catheter removal was not described. There were no neurologic complications. While the results of this study are reassuring, the obsolescence of the thrombotest as a measure of anticoagulation combined with the unknown coagulation status of the patients at the time of catheter removal limit their usefulness.

The use of an in-dwelling epidural or intrathecal catheter and the timing of its removal in an anticoagulated patient are also controversial. Although the trauma of needle placement occurs with both single dose and continuous catheter techniques, the presence of an in-dwelling catheter could theoretically provoke additional injury to tissue and vascular structures. There were no reported spinal hematomas in 192 patients receiving postoperative epidural analgesia in conjunction with low-dose warfarin after total knee arthroplasty. Patients received warfarin to prolong the PT to 15.0 to 17.3 seconds (normal 10.9–12.8 seconds), corresponding to an international normalized ratio (INR) of 2.0 to 3.0. Epidural catheters were left in-dwelling 37 ±15 hours (range 13–96 hours). Mean PT at the time of epidural catheter removal was 13.4 ± 2 seconds (range 10.6–25.8 seconds). This study documents the relative safety of low-dose warfarin anticoagulation in patients with an in-dwelling epidural catheter. However, there was a large variability in patient response to warfarin, and the authors recommended close monitoring of coagulation status to avoid excessive prolongation of the PT (32). There were also no neurologic complications among 459 orthopedic patients studied by Wu and Perkins (33) who underwent spinal or epidural anesthesia, including 412 patients who received postoperative epidural analgesia. All patients were anticoagulated with warfarin postoperatively; 181 patients also received a warfarin dose preoperatively. Mean duration of epidural analgesia was 43.6 ± 12.5 hours. Patients who had warfarin prophylaxis administered preoperatively had significantly higher PTs at the time of catheter removal.

Regional Anesthetic Management of the Patient on Oral Anticoagulants

Anesthetic management of patients anticoagulated perioperatively with warfarin is dependent on dosage and timing of initiation of therapy. The PT and INR of patients on chronic oral anticoagulation will require 3 to 5 days to normalize after discontinuation of the anticoagulant therapy. Theoretically, since the PT and INR reflect predominantly factor VII activity (and factor VII has only a 6- to 8-hour half-life), there may be an interval during which the PT and INR approach normal values, yet factors II and X levels may not be adequate for normal hemostasis. Therefore, it is recommended that documentation of the patient's normal coagulation status be achieved prior to implementation of neuraxial block (10).

Many orthopedic surgeons administer the first dose of warfarin the night before surgery. For these patients, the PT and INR should be checked prior to neuraxial block if the first dose was given more than 24 hours earlier or a second dose of oral anticoagulant has been administered. Patients receiving low-dose warfarin therapy during epidural analgesia should have their PT and INR monitored on a daily basis and checked before catheter removal, if initial dose of warfarin was more than 36 hours beforehand. Initial studies evaluating the safety of epidural analgesia in association with oral anticoagulation utilized low-dose warfarin, with the mean daily doses of approximately 5 mg. Higher doses of warfarin may require more intensive monitoring of the coagulation status. Reduced doses of warfarin should be given to patients who are likely to have an enhanced response to the drug (10). An INR > 3 should prompt the physician to withhold or reduce the warfarin dose in patients with in-dwelling neuraxial catheters. There is no definitive recommendation for removal of neuraxial catheters in patients with therapeutic levels of anticoagulation during a neuraxial catheter infusion. Caution must be exercised in making decisions about removing or maintaining these catheters (10).

Thrombolytic and Fibrinolytic Therapy

Thrombolytic agents actively dissolve fibrin clots that have already formed. Exogenous plasminogen activators, such as streptokinase and urokinase, not only dissolve thrombus but also affect circulating plasminogen as well, leading to decreased levels of both plasminogen and fibrin. Recombinant tissue-type plasminogen activator (rt-PA), an endogenous agent, is more fibrin-selective and has less effect on circulating plasminogen levels (34). Clot lysis leads to elevation of fibrin degradation products, which themselves have an anticoagulant effect by inhibiting platelet aggregation. In addition to the fibrinolytic agent, these patients frequently receive intravenous heparin to maintain an APTT of 1.5 to 2 times normal (35).

In an initial study involving 290 patients with acute myocardial infarction who were treated with thrombolytic therapy (streptokinase or rt-PA) and subsequently heparinized, fibrinogen and plasminogen were maximally depressed at 5 hours after thrombolytic therapy and remain significantly depressed at 27 hours. Although the decrease in coagulation factor levels was greater with streptokinase therapy, the frequency of hemorrhagic events was similar between patient groups; 33% of the rt-PA patients and 31% of the streptokinase patients. For more than 70% of the patients with hemorrhagic events in each group, the primary bleeding site was the catheterization or other puncture site. The authors recommended avoiding invasive procedures in patients receiving thrombolytic therapy (35).

While epidural or spinal needle and catheter placement with subsequent heparinization appears relatively safe, the risk of spinal hematoma in patients who receive thrombolytic therapy is less well defined. No controlled studies have examined the risk. Several cases of spinal hematoma in patients with in-dwelling epidural catheters who received thrombolytic agents have been reported in the literature. Dickman et al. (36) reported a case in which a patient with femoral artery occlusion received an epidural anesthetic for surgical placement of an intra-arterial catheter for infusion of urokinase. Three hours postoperatively, the patient complained of back pain, which progressed to paraplegia despite discontinuation of the urokinase infusion. An emergency decompressive laminectomy was performed, and a large solidified hematoma compressing the thecal sac was evacuated. The patient recovered full neurologic function within 3 days. Onishchuk and Carlsson (37) reported a patient with superficial femoral artery occlusion who underwent epidural catheter placement for femoral-popliteal artery bypass. Blood was noted in the epidural catheter during placement. The patient was bolused with 6,300 U of heparin 90 minutes later, and a single bolus of urokinase was also injected intra-arterially during the surgical procedure. A heparin infusion of 1,000 U/h was initiated and continued postoperatively for 24 hours. The patient was taken to the recovery room and the epidural catheter removed. On the fourth postoperative day, it was noted the patient developed paraplegia. An MRI revealed an epidural hematoma extending from T10-L2. An emergency decompressive laminectomy was performed without any improvement. The authors recommended that epidural anesthesia be avoided in patients who will receive thrombolytic therapy.

Regional Anesthetic Management of the Patient on Thrombolytics and Fibrinolytics

The physiologic state induced by the use of fibrinolytic and thrombolytic agents represents a unique problem in the performance of regional anesthesia. Patients receiving concurrent heparin with fibrinolytic and thrombolytic drugs are at high risk of adverse neuraxial bleeding during spinal or epidural anesthesia (11).

Patients receiving fibrinolytic and thrombolytic drugs should be cautioned against receiving spinal or epidural anesthetics except in highly unusual circumstances. Guidelines detailing original contraindications for thrombolytic drugs suggest avoidance of these drugs within 10 days of puncture of noncompressible vessels. Data are not available to clearly outline the length of time neuraxial puncture should be avoided after discontinuation of these drugs (11).

Neurologic monitoring needs to be carried out for an appropriate interval. It may be that the interval of monitoring should not be more than 2 hours between neurologic checks. Furthermore, if neuraxial blocks have been combined with fibrinolytic and thrombolytic therapy and ongoing epidural catheter infusion, the infusion should be limited to drugs minimizing sensory and motor blockade (11).

There is no definitive recommendation for removal of neuraxial catheters in patients who unexpectedly receive fibrinolytic and thrombolytic therapy during a neuraxial catheter infusion. Caution must be exercised in making decisions about removing or maintaining these catheters. The measurement of fibrinogen may be helpful in making a decision about catheter removal or maintenance (11).

Antiplatelet Therapy

Antiplatelet therapy, including such medications as aspirin, naproxen, piroxicam, and ketorolac, has been considered a relative contraindication to central neural blockade by some authors due to the associated prolongation of the bleeding time and theoretically greater risk of spinal hematoma formation.

Antiplatelet medications inhibit platelet cyclooxygenase and prevent the synthesis of thromboxane A_2. Thromboxane A_2 is not only a potent vasoconstrictor, but also facilitates secondary platelet aggregation and release reactions. Platelets from patients who have been taking these medications have normal platelet adherence to subendothelium and normal primary hemostatic plug formation. Thus an adequate, although potentially fragile, clot may form. While such plugs may be satisfactory hemostatic barriers for smaller vascular lesions, they may not ensure adequate perioperative hemostatic clot formation.

Ticlopidine and clopidogrel are also platelet aggregation inhibitors. These antiplatelet agents, used in the prevention of cerebrovascular thromboembolic events, effect both primary *and* secondary platelet aggregation. Ticlopidine and clopidogrel also interfere with platelet-fibrinogen binding and subsequent platelet-platelet interactions. The effects are irreversible and present for the life of the platelet. Since ticlopidine and clopidogrel act independently of aspirin, they have no effect on platelet cyclooxygenase. However, it is important to note that these new platelet aggregation inhibitors and aspirin have not been tested in combination and drug labeling recommends against concomitant administration. There have been two reported spinal hematomas with these agents (38, 39).

Abciximab (Reopro®) also inhibits platelet aggregation through binding to the platelet glycoprotein IIb/ IIIa receptor. Abciximab additionally binds to the vibronectin receptor found on platelets and vessel wall endothelial cells. Platelet function generally recovers over 48 hours. However, the drug remains in the circulation 15 days or more bound to platelets. Abciximab is indicated as an adjunct to percutaneous coronary intervention and in patients with unstable angina (when percutaneous coronary intervention is planned within 24 hours) and is administered in combination with aspirin and heparin. The profound effects on the hemostatic system following this treatment regimen (abciximab, heparin, and aspirin) precludes the performance of neuraxial techniques. Likewise, the pharmacologic differences between ticlopidine/clopidogrel and the aspirin-type antiplatelet agents makes it impossible to extrapolate between the two groups of drugs regarding the practice of regional anesthesia. Subsequent discussion pertains to antiplatelet agents affecting secondary platelet reactions only.

It has been suggested that the Ivy bleeding time is the most reliable predictor of abnormal bleeding in patients receiving antiplatelet drugs. However, the "postaspirin" bleeding time is not a reliable indicator of platelet function (40, 41). Although the bleeding time may normalize within 3 days after aspirin ingestion, platelet function as measured by platelet response to adenosine diphosphate, epinephrine, and collagen may take a week to return to normal. There is no evidence to suggest that a bleeding time can predict hemostatic compromise; studies have failed to show a correlation between aspirin-induced prolongation of the bleeding time and surgical blood loss (40). Therefore, measurement of an Ivy bleeding time before induction of spinal or epidural anesthesia may not identify those patients at increased risk for hemorrhagic complications and is clinically not indicated. Other nonsteroidal analgesics (naproxen, piroxicam, ibuprofen) produce a short-term defect that normalizes within 3 days (42). Platelet function in patients receiving antiplatelet medications should be assumed to be decreased for 1 week with aspirin and 1 to 3 days with other nonsteroidal anti-inflammatory drugs. Special platelet function assays are also available to monitor platelet aggregation and degranulation.

There has been a single reported case of spontaneous epidural hematoma formation (in the absence of spinal or epidural anesthesia) in a patient with a history of aspirin ingestion (43). The patient self-administered 1,500 mg of aspirin in the form of an aspirin-containing antacid and a short time later complained of severe lower extremity weakness. A myelogram revealed complete epidural block at T5–6 level. The cerebrospinal fluid was clear, although prolonged bleeding from the lumbar puncture site was noted after myelography. A laminectomy was performed and the hematoma removed. Neurologic function gradually improved.

The risk associated with administration of spinal or epidural anesthesia to a patient receiving antiplatelet medications remains controversial. Although Vandermeulen et al. (18) implicated antiplatelet therapy in 3 of the 61 cases of spinal hematoma occurring after spinal or epidural anesthesia, several large studies have demonstrated the relative safety of central neural blockade in combination with antiplatelet therapy. The Collaborative Low-dose Aspirin Study in Pregnancy (CLASP) Group included 1,422 high-risk obstetric patients administered 60 mg aspirin daily who underwent epidural anesthesia without any neurologic sequelae. However, no data regarding difficulty or bleeding during epidural needle or catheter was reported (3). Horlocker et al. (44) retrospectively reported 1,013 spinal and epidural anesthetics in which antiplatelet drugs were taken by 39% of the patients, including 11% of patients who were on multiple antiplatelet medications. While no patient developed signs of spinal hematoma, patients on antiplatelet medications showed a higher incidence of blood aspirated through the spinal or epidural needle or catheter.

This study was subsequently performed prospectively on an additional 1,000 patients, 39% of whom reported preoperative antiplatelet therapy (45). As before, there were no spinal hematomas. Blood was noted during needle or catheter placement in 22% of patients, including 7% of patients with frank blood. Preoperative antiplatelet therapy was not a risk factor for bloody needle or catheter placement. However, many patient and anesthetic variables including female gender, increased age, a history of excessive bruising or bleeding, continuous catheter technique, large needle gauge, multiple needle passes, and difficult needle placement were significant risk factors. The lack of correlation between antiplatelet medications and bloody needle or catheter placement (producing clinically insignificant collections of blood within the spinal canal) is strong evidence that preoperative antiplatelet therapy is not a significant risk factor for the development of neurologic dysfunction from spinal hematoma in patients who undergo spinal or epidural anesthesia while receiving these medications.

Regional Anesthetic Management of the Patient Receiving Antiplatelet Medications

Antiplatelet drugs, by themselves, appear to represent no added significant risk for the development of spinal hematoma in patients having epidural or spinal anesthesia. However, the concurrent use of medications that affect other components of the clotting mechanisms, such as oral anticoagulants, standard heparin, and LMWH, may increase the risk of bleeding complications for patients receiving antiplatelet agents. Assessment of platelet function prior to performance of neuraxial block is not recommended. However, careful preoperative assessment of the patient to identify alterations of health that might contribute to bleeding is crucial (12). Since the risk of spinal bleeding associated with ticlopidine and clopidogrel is unknown (but theoretically greater than aspirin-like drugs), clinicians should proceed cautiously.

CONCLUSION

In summary, the decision to perform spinal or epidural anesthesia/ analgesia and the timing of catheter removal in a patient receiving

TABLE 8–3. Pharmacologic Activities of Anticoagulants, Antiplatelet Agents and Thrombolytics

Agent	Effect On Coagulation Variables		Peak Effect	Time to Normal Time To Discontinuation	Comments Hemostasis after
	PT	aPTT			
Intravenous Heparin	↑	↑↑↑	Minutes	4–6 hours	Monitor ACT, aPTT, delay heparinization for 1 hour after needle placement.
Subcutaneous Heparin	—	↑	40–50 minutes	4–6 hours	APTT may remain normal, anti-Xa activity reflects degree of anticoagulation.
Low Molecular Weight Heparin	—	—	3–5 hours	12–24 hours	Anti-Xa activity not monitored. Use with caution in patients receiving epidural analgesia
Warfarin	↑↑↑	↑	4–6 days (Less with loading dose)	4–6 days	Monitor PT daily, remove in-dwelling neuraxial catheter when INR < 1.5.
Antiplatelet Agents Aspirin Other NSAID Glycoprotein IIb/IIIa receptor inhibitors	—	—	Hours	5–8 days 1–3 days 1–2 weeks	Bleeding time not reliable predictor of platelet function. No increased risk with NSAIDs; risk associated with ticlopidine, clopidogrel and other IIb/IIIa inhibitors unknown
Fibrinolytics	↑	↑↑	Minutes	24–36 hours	Fibrinogen level decreased for 1–2 days. Heparin administered in combination. Neuraxial block not recommended.

PT = Prothrombin time; aPTT = Activated partial thromboplastin time; ACT = Activated clotting time; ↑ = Clinically insignificant increase; ↑↑ = Possibly clinically significant increase; ↑↑↑ = Clinically significant increase; NSAID = Nonsteroidal anti-inflammatory drug thromboprophylaxis should be made on an individual basis, weighing the small, though definite risk of spinal hematoma with the benefits of regional anesthesia for a specific patient. Alternative anesthetic and analgesic techniques exist for patients considered to be at an unacceptable risk. The patient's coagulation status should be optimized at the time of spinal or epidural needle/catheter placement, and the level of anticoagulation must be carefully monitored during the period of epidural catheterization. It is important to note that patients respond with variable sensitivities to anticoagulant medications (Table 9–3). In-dwelling catheters should not be removed in the presence of therapeutic anticoagulation, as this appears to significantly increase the risk of spinal hematoma. In addition, communication between clinicians involved in the perioperative management of patients receiving anticoagulants for thromboprophylaxis is essential in order to decrease the risk of serious hemorrhagic complications. Patients should be monitored closely in the perioperative period for early signs of cord compression. If spinal hematoma is suspected, the treatment of choice is immediate decompressive laminectomy. Recovery is unlikely if surgery is postponed for more than 8 to 12 hours; less than 40% of the patients in Vandermeulen's series had partial or good recovery of neurologic function (18).

References

1. Usubiaga JE: Neurologic complications following epidural anesthesia. Int Anesthesiol Clin 13:1–153, 1975
2. Bonica JJ: The Management of Pain. 1st ed. Philadelphia: Lea and Febiger, 1953
3. CLASP (Collaborative Low-Dose Aspirin Study in Pregnancy) Collaborative Group: CLASP: A randomized trial of low-dose aspirin for the prevention and treatment of pre-eclampsia among 9364 pregnant women. Lancet 343:619–629, 1994
4. Odoom JA, Sih IL: Epidural analgesia and anticoagulant therapy. Anaesthesia 38:254–259, 1983
5. Rao TLK, El-Etr AA: Anticoagulation following placement of epidural and subarachnoid catheters: An evaluation of neurologic sequelae. Anesthesiology 55:618–620, 1981
6. Bergqvist D, Lindblad B, Mätzsch T: Low molecular weight heparin for thromboprophylaxis and epidural/spinal anaesthesia: Is there a risk? Acta Anaesthesiol Scand 36:605–609, 1992
7. Schwander D, Bachmann F: Heparine et anesthesies medullaires: analyse de decision. Ann Fr Anesth Reanim 10:284–296, 1991
8. Liu SS, Mulroy MF: Neuraxial anesthesia and analgesia in the presence of standard heparin. Reg Anesth Pain Med 23:157–163, 1998

9. Horlocker TT, Wedel DJ: Neuraxial block and low molecular weight heparin: Balancing perioperative analgesia and thrombo-prophylaxis. Reg Anesth Pain Med 23:164–177, 1998

10. Enneking KF, Benzon HT: Oral anticoagulants and regional anesthesia: A perspective. Reg Anesth Pain Med 23:140–145, 1998

11. Rosenquist RW, Brown DL: Neuraxial bleeding: Fibrinolytics/thrombolytics. Reg Anesth Pain Med 23:152–156, 1998

12. Urmey WF, Rowlingson JC: Do antiplatelet agents contribute to the development of perioperative spinal hematoma? Reg Anesth Pain Med 23:146–151, 1998

13. Liu S, Carpenter RL, Neal JM: Epidural anesthesia and analgesia. Their role in postoperative outcome. Anesthesiology 82:1474–1506, 1995

14. Tuman KJ, McCarthy RJ, March RJ, et al: Effects of epidural anesthesia and analgesia on coagulation and outcome after major vascular surgery. Anesth Analg 73:696–704, 1991

15. Chaney MA: Intrathecal and epidural anesthesia and analgesia for cardiac surgery. Anesth Analg 84:1211–1221, 1997

16. Tryba M: Rückmarksnahe regionalanästhesie und niedermolekulare heparine: Pro. Anästh Intensivmed Notfallmed Schmerzther 28:179–181, 1993

17. Spurny OM, Rubin S, Wolff JW, et al: Spinal epidural hematoma during anticoagulant therapy. Arch Intern Med 114:103–107, 1964

18. Vandermeulen EP, Van Aken H, Vermylen J: Anticoagulants and spinal-epidural anesthesia. Anesth Analg 79:1165–1177, 1994

19. Baron HC, LaRaja RD, Rossi G, Atkinson D: Continuous epidural analgesia in the heparinized vascular surgical patient: A retrospective review of 912 patients. J Vasc Surg 6:144–146, 1987

20. Mathews ET, Abrams LD: Intrathecal morphine in open heart surgery (letter). Lancet 2:543, 1980

21. Cheney FW, Domino KB, Caplan RA, Posner KL: Nerve injury associated with anesthesia. A closed claims analysis. Anesthesiology 90:1062–1069, 1999

22. Goldstein S, Dean D, Kim SJ, Cocozell K, Grofsik J, Silver P, Cody RP: A survey of spinal and epidural techniques in adult cardiac surgery. J Cardiothorac Vasc Anesth 15:158–168, 2001

23. Ruff RL, Dougherty JH: Complications of lumbar puncture followed by anticoagulation. Stroke 12:879–881, 1981

24. Poller L, Taberner DA, Sandilands DG, Galasko CSB: An evaluation of APTT monitoring of low-dose heparin dosage in hip surgery. Thromb Haemostas 47:50–53, 1982

25. Lowson SM, Goodchild CS: Low-dose heparin therapy and spinal anesthesia. Anaesthesia 44:67–68, 1989

26. Allemann BH, Gerber H, Gruber UF: Rückenmarksnahe anaesthe-

sie und subkutan verabreichtes low-dose heparin-dihydergot zur thromboembolieprophylaxe. Anaesthetist 32:80–83, 1983

27. Darnat S, Guggiari M, Grob R, et al: Un cas d'hematome extradural rachidien au cours de la mise en place d'un catheter peridural. Ann Fr Anesth Reanim 5:550–552, 1986

28. Dupeyrat A, Dequire PM, Merouani A, et al: Hematome sous-arachnoidien et rachianesthesie. Ann Fr Anesth Reanim 9:560–562, 1990

29. Metzger G, Singbartl G: Spinal epidural hematoma following epidural anesthesia versus spontaneous spinal subdural hematoma. Two case reports. Acta Anaesthesiol Scand 35:105–107, 1991

30. Hirsh J, Levine MN: Low molecular weight heparin: Laboratory properties and clinical evaluation. Eur J Surg 571(Suppl):9–22, 1994

31. Schroeder DR: Statistics: Detecting a rare adverse drug reaction using spontaneous reports. Reg Anesth Pain Med 23:183–189, 1998

32. Horlocker TT, Wedel DJ, Schlichting JL: Postoperative epidural analgesia and oral anticoagulant therapy. Anesth Analg 79:89–93, 1994

33. Wu C, Perkins FM: Oral anticoagulant prophylaxis and epidural catheter removal. Reg Anesth 21:503–507, 1996

34. Hirsch DR, Goldhaber SZ: Bleeding time and other laboratory tests to monitor the safety and efficacy of thrombolytic therapy. Chest 97:124S–131S, 1990

35. Rao AK, Pratt C, Berke A, et al: Thrombolysis in myocardial infarction trial—Phase I: Hemorrhagic manifestations and changes in plasma fibrinogen and the fibrinolytic system in patients treated with recombinant tissue plasminogen activator and streptokinase. J Am Coll Cardiol 11:1–11, 1988

36. Dickman CA, Shedd SA, Spetzler RF, et al: Spinal epidural hematoma associated with epidural anesthesia: Complications of systemic heparinization in patients receiving peripheral vascular thrombolytic therapy. Anesthesiology 72:947–950, 1990

37. Onishchuk JL, Carlsson C: Epidural hematoma associated with epidural anesthesia: Complications of anticoagulant therapy. Anesthesiology 77:1221–1223, 1992

38. Mayumi T, Dohi S: Spinal subarachnoid hematoma after lumbar puncture in a patient receiving antiplatelet therapy. Anesth Analg 62:777–779, 1983

39. Benzon HT, Wong HY, Siddiqui T, Ondra S: Caution in performing epidural injections in patients on several antiplatelet drugs. Anesthesiology 91:1558–1559, 1999

40. Rodgers RPC, Levin J: A critical reappraisal of the bleeding time. Semin Thromb Hemost 16:1–20, 1990

41. Hindman BJ, Koka BV: Usefulness of the post-aspirin bleeding time. Anesthesiology 64:368–370, 1986
42. Cronberg S, Wallmark E, Soderberg I: Effect on platelet aggregation of oral administration of 10 non-steroidal analgesics to humans. Scand J Haematol 33:155–159, 1984
43. Locke GE, Giorgio AJ, Biggers SL, et al: Acute spinal epidural hematoma secondary to aspirin-induced prolonged bleeding. Surg Neurol 5:293–296, 1976
44. Horlocker TT, Wedel DJ, Offord KP: Does preoperative antiplatelet therapy increase the risk of hemorrhagic complications associated with regional anesthesia? Anesth Analg 70:631–634, 1990
45. Horlocker TT, Wedel DJ, Offord KP, et al: Preoperative antiplatelet therapy does not increase the risk of spinal hematoma associated with regional anesthesia. Anesth Analg 80:303–309, 1995

Index

NOTE: Figures indicated by italic numbers; Tables indicated by t

Arrhythmias
post-thoracotomy, TEA and,
125–126
Aspirin, 155

β-Blockers
EPI local anesthetics and, 70
TEA and, 25
Bezold-Jarisch reflex
bradycardia, LEA and TEA, 27
Bradycardia
Bezold-Jarisch reflex, LEA and
TEA, 27
Bupivacaine, 1–2
epidural intraoperative, 66
liposomal delivery, 9
polyester microspheres, 9–10
for TEA, 126–127

Cardiac surgery
adult
epidural techniques, 59–79
intrathecal techniques for,
39–57
neonatal, intense analgesia and,
40
pediatric
epidural techniques, 103–105
intrathecal techniques,
102–103
regional anesthesia for, 97–110
Cardiopulmonary bypass grafting
(CABG)
epidural analgesia and, 67
intense analgesia and, 40, 60
stress-response hormones and,
40
Cardiotoxicity
bupivacaine, 2
levobupivacaine, 5–7, 7t
lidocaine, 2–3
ropivacaine, 2–3, 6–7, 7t
Cardiovascular depression
LEA and TEA, 27
Cerebral blood flow, 21
Chronic obstructive pulmonary
disease
endoTAAR use in, 92
Circulatory stability
regional anesthesia in pediatric
cardiac surgery, 98–99
Clopidogrel, 155
Coagulopathies

pre-existing, risk for hemorrhage,
139
Cold pressor test (CPT), 22, *22*
Coumarin
regional anesthesia and anticoagulation, 140
Cryoanalgesia
use in thoracotomy, 116

Depo-morphine, 8–9

Endoleak
in AAA repair, 85–86
Endothelium
sympathetic activity and, 23
Endovascular abdominal aortic
aneurysm repair
(endoAAAR), 81
anticoagulation management, 93
chronic obstructive pulmonary
disease, 92
goals for anesthesia in, 89
intraoperative complications,
89–92
local sedation techniques for,
92
Endovascular aortic grafts
endoleak, 85–86
final angiogram after deployment, *88*
follow-up, 87–88
goals for anesthesia in, 89
initial reports, 83
long-term patency and durability,
88–89
major complications, 85
managing intraoperative complications, 89–92
misdeployment, 90
positioning, *86–87*
preimplantation calibrated
angiography, 84
rupture, 90
setting for performance of, 87
technique for implantation, 84
Endovascular procedures
regional anesthesia for, 81–96
Endovascular Technologies (EVT)
device
AAA repair, 83
Endovascular thoracoabdominal
aortic aneurysm repair
(endoTAAR), 91